# THIS BOOK BELONGS TO:

| CONTACT INFORMATION | |
|---|---|
| NAME: | |
| ADDRESS: | |
| PHONE: | |

START / END DATES

___ / ___ / ___    TO    ___ / ___ / ___

# DEDICATION

This Mood Tracker Journal Log book is dedicated to all the people out there who want to record their moods and document their findings in the process.

You are my inspiration for producing books and I'm honored to be a part of keeping all of your mood notes and records organized.

This journal notebook will help you record your details about your mood.

Thoughtfully put together with these sections to record:

Date, Month, & Week, Happy, Neutral, or Sad, Emotion, What Happened, and Daily Score.

# HOW TO USE THIS BOOK

The purpose of this book is to keep all of your Mood notes all in one place. It will help keep you organized.

This Mood Tracker Journal will allow you to accurately document every detail about your mood. It's a great way to chart your course through finding mood balance.

Here are examples of the prompts for you to fill in and write about your experience in this book:

1. **Date, Month & Week** - For writing the date, which month, and the week of.

2. **Happy, Neutral, or Sad** - Each day you can record for the morning, the afternoon, and the evening whether you were mostly happy, neutral, or sad.

3. **Emotion** - Log the emotion that you felt.

4. **What Happened** - Write your notes on what happened to give you that emotion, any gratitude you have, any symptoms, quotes for the day, things that happened, your energy, any feeling you experience, any pain medication you take, etc.

5. **Daily Score** - Rate your mood level for your overall day, from 1-5 stars.

# Mood Tracker

| MONTH | | | | | WEEK | | |
|---|---|---|---|---|---|---|---|

| | MONDAY | TUESDAY | WEDNESDAY | THURSDAY | FRIDAY | SATURDAY | SUNDAY |
|---|---|---|---|---|---|---|---|
| HAPPY | | | | | | | |
| NEUTRAL | | | | | | | |
| SAD | | | | | | | |

| DAY | EMOTION | WHAT HAPPENED? | DAILY SCORE |
|---|---|---|---|
| MONDAY | | | ☆ ☆ ☆ ☆ ☆ |
| TUESDAY | | | ☆ ☆ ☆ ☆ ☆ |
| WEDNESDAY | | | ☆ ☆ ☆ ☆ ☆ |
| THURSDAY | | | ☆ ☆ ☆ ☆ ☆ |
| FRIDAY | | | ☆ ☆ ☆ ☆ ☆ |
| SATURDAY | | | ☆ ☆ ☆ ☆ ☆ |
| SUNDAY | | | ☆ ☆ ☆ ☆ ☆ |

# Mood Tracker

| MONTH | | | | | WEEK | | | |
|---|---|---|---|---|---|---|---|---|

| | MONDAY | TUESDAY | WEDNESDAY | THURSDAY | FRIDAY | SATURDAY | SUNDAY |
|---|---|---|---|---|---|---|---|
| HAPPY | | | | | | | |
| NEUTRAL | | | | | | | |
| SAD | | | | | | | |

| DAY | EMOTION | WHAT HAPPENED? | DAILY SCORE |
|---|---|---|---|
| MONDAY | | | ☆ ☆ ☆ ☆ ☆ |
| TUESDAY | | | ☆ ☆ ☆ ☆ ☆ |
| WEDNESDAY | | | ☆ ☆ ☆ ☆ ☆ |
| THURSDAY | | | ☆ ☆ ☆ ☆ ☆ |
| FRIDAY | | | ☆ ☆ ☆ ☆ ☆ |
| SATURDAY | | | ☆ ☆ ☆ ☆ ☆ |
| SUNDAY | | | ☆ ☆ ☆ ☆ ☆ |

# Mood Tracker

| MONTH | | WEEK | |
|-------|---|------|---|

| | MONDAY | TUESDAY | WEDNESDAY | THURSDAY | FRIDAY | SATURDAY | SUNDAY |
|---------|--------|---------|-----------|----------|--------|----------|--------|
| HAPPY | | | | | | | |
| NEUTRAL | | | | | | | |
| SAD | | | | | | | |

| DAY | EMOTION | WHAT HAPPENED? | DAILY SCORE |
|-----|---------|----------------|-------------|
| MONDAY | | | ☆ ☆ ☆ ☆ ☆ |
| TUESDAY | | | ☆ ☆ ☆ ☆ ☆ |
| WEDNESDAY | | | ☆ ☆ ☆ ☆ ☆ |
| THURSDAY | | | ☆ ☆ ☆ ☆ ☆ |
| FRIDAY | | | ☆ ☆ ☆ ☆ ☆ |
| SATURDAY | | | ☆ ☆ ☆ ☆ ☆ |
| SUNDAY | | | ☆ ☆ ☆ ☆ ☆ |

# Mood Tracker

| MONTH | | | | | | | | WEEK | | |
|-------|---|---|---|---|---|---|---|------|---|---|

| | MONDAY | TUESDAY | WEDNESDAY | THURSDAY | FRIDAY | SATURDAY | SUNDAY |
|-------|--------|---------|-----------|----------|--------|----------|--------|
| HAPPY | | | | | | | |
| NEUTRAL | | | | | | | |
| SAD | | | | | | | |

| DAY | EMOTION | WHAT HAPPENED? | DAILY SCORE |
|-----|---------|----------------|-------------|
| MONDAY | | | ☆ ☆ ☆ ☆ ☆ |
| TUESDAY | | | ☆ ☆ ☆ ☆ ☆ |
| WEDNESDAY | | | ☆ ☆ ☆ ☆ ☆ |
| THURSDAY | | | ☆ ☆ ☆ ☆ ☆ |
| FRIDAY | | | ☆ ☆ ☆ ☆ ☆ |
| SATURDAY | | | ☆ ☆ ☆ ☆ ☆ |
| SUNDAY | | | ☆ ☆ ☆ ☆ ☆ |

# Mood Tracker

| MONTH | | WEEK | |
|---|---|---|---|

| | MONDAY | TUESDAY | WEDNESDAY | THURSDAY | FRIDAY | SATURDAY | SUNDAY |
|---|---|---|---|---|---|---|---|
| HAPPY | | | | | | | |
| NEUTRAL | | | | | | | |
| SAD | | | | | | | |

| DAY | EMOTION | WHAT HAPPENED? | DAILY SCORE |
|---|---|---|---|
| MONDAY | | | ☆ ☆ ☆ ☆ ☆ |
| TUESDAY | | | ☆ ☆ ☆ ☆ ☆ |
| WEDNESDAY | | | ☆ ☆ ☆ ☆ ☆ |
| THURSDAY | | | ★ ★ ★ ★ ★ |
| FRIDAY | | | ☆ ☆ ☆ ☆ ☆ |
| SATURDAY | | | ☆ ☆ ☆ ☆ ☆ |
| SUNDAY | | | ☆ ☆ ☆ ☆ ☆ |

# Mood Tracker

| MONTH | | | | | | | WEEK | | |
|---|---|---|---|---|---|---|---|---|---|

| | MONDAY | TUESDAY | WEDNESDAY | THURSDAY | FRIDAY | SATURDAY | SUNDAY |
|---|---|---|---|---|---|---|---|
| **HAPPY** | | | | | | | |
| **NEUTRAL** | | | | | | | |
| **SAD** | | | | | | | |

| DAY | EMOTION | WHAT HAPPENED? | DAILY SCORE |
|---|---|---|---|
| MONDAY | | | ☆ ☆ ☆ ☆ ☆ |
| TUESDAY | | | ☆ ☆ ☆ ☆ ☆ |
| WEDNESDAY | | | ☆ ☆ ☆ ☆ ☆ |
| THURSDAY | | | ☆ ☆ ☆ ☆ ☆ |
| FRIDAY | | | ☆ ☆ ☆ ☆ ☆ |
| SATURDAY | | | ☆ ☆ ☆ ☆ ☆ |
| SUNDAY | | | ☆ ☆ ☆ ☆ ☆ |

# Mood Tracker

| MONTH | | | WEEK | |

| | MONDAY | TUESDAY | WEDNESDAY | THURSDAY | FRIDAY | SATURDAY | SUNDAY |
|---|---|---|---|---|---|---|---|
| HAPPY | | | | | | | |
| NEUTRAL | | | | | | | |
| SAD | | | | | | | |

| DAY | EMOTION | WHAT HAPPENED? | DAILY SCORE |
|---|---|---|---|
| MONDAY | | | ☆ ☆ ☆ ☆ ☆ |
| TUESDAY | | | ☆ ☆ ☆ ☆ ☆ |
| WEDNESDAY | | | ☆ ☆ ☆ ☆ ☆ |
| THURSDAY | | | ☆ ☆ ☆ ☆ ☆ |
| FRIDAY | | | ☆ ☆ ☆ ☆ ☆ |
| SATURDAY | | | ☆ ☆ ☆ ☆ ☆ |
| SUNDAY | | | ☆ ☆ ☆ ☆ ☆ |

# Mood Tracker

| MONTH | | | | | | WEEK | | | | |
|---|---|---|---|---|---|---|---|---|---|---|

| | MONDAY | TUESDAY | WEDNESDAY | THURSDAY | FRIDAY | SATURDAY | SUNDAY |
|---|---|---|---|---|---|---|---|
| HAPPY | | | | | | | |
| NEUTRAL | | | | | | | |
| SAD | | | | | | | |

| DAY | EMOTION | WHAT HAPPENED? | DAILY SCORE |
|---|---|---|---|
| MONDAY | | | ☆ ☆ ☆ ☆ ☆ |
| TUESDAY | | | ☆ ☆ ☆ ☆ ☆ |
| WEDNESDAY | | | ☆ ☆ ☆ ☆ ☆ |
| THURSDAY | | | ☆ ☆ ☆ ☆ ☆ |
| FRIDAY | | | ☆ ☆ ☆ ☆ ☆ |
| SATURDAY | | | ☆ ☆ ☆ ☆ ☆ |
| SUNDAY | | | ☆ ☆ ☆ ☆ ☆ |

# Mood Tracker

| MONTH | | | | | | WEEK | | | |
|---|---|---|---|---|---|---|---|---|---|

| | MONDAY | TUESDAY | WEDNESDAY | THURSDAY | FRIDAY | SATURDAY | SUNDAY |
|---|---|---|---|---|---|---|---|
| HAPPY | | | | | | | |
| NEUTRAL | | | | | | | |
| SAD | | | | | | | |

| DAY | EMOTION | WHAT HAPPENED? | DAILY SCORE |
|---|---|---|---|
| MONDAY | | | ☆ ☆ ☆ ☆ ☆ |
| TUESDAY | | | ☆ ☆ ☆ ☆ ☆ |
| WEDNESDAY | | | ☆ ☆ ☆ ☆ ☆ |
| THURSDAY | | | ☆ ☆ ☆ ☆ ☆ |
| FRIDAY | | | ☆ ☆ ☆ ☆ ☆ |
| SATURDAY | | | ☆ ☆ ☆ ☆ ☆ |
| SUNDAY | | | ☆ ☆ ☆ ☆ ☆ |

# Mood Tracker

| MONTH | | | | | | | WEEK | | |
|---|---|---|---|---|---|---|---|---|---|

| | MONDAY | TUESDAY | WEDNESDAY | THURSDAY | FRIDAY | SATURDAY | SUNDAY |
|---|---|---|---|---|---|---|---|
| HAPPY | | | | | | | |
| NEUTRAL | | | | | | | |
| SAD | | | | | | | |

| DAY | EMOTION | WHAT HAPPENED? | DAILY SCORE |
|---|---|---|---|
| MONDAY | | | ☆ ☆ ☆ ☆ ☆ |
| TUESDAY | | | ☆ ☆ ☆ ☆ ☆ |
| WEDNESDAY | | | ☆ ☆ ☆ ☆ ☆ |
| THURSDAY | | | ☆ ☆ ☆ ☆ ☆ |
| FRIDAY | | | ☆ ☆ ☆ ☆ ☆ |
| SATURDAY | | | ☆ ☆ ☆ ☆ ☆ |
| SUNDAY | | | ☆ ☆ ☆ ☆ ☆ |

# Mood Tracker

| MONTH | | | | | | WEEK | | |
|-------|--|--|--|--|--|------|--|--|

| | MONDAY | TUESDAY | WEDNESDAY | THURSDAY | FRIDAY | SATURDAY | SUNDAY |
|-------|--------|---------|-----------|----------|--------|----------|--------|
| HAPPY | | | | | | | |
| NEUTRAL | | | | | | | |
| SAD | | | | | | | |

| DAY | EMOTION | WHAT HAPPENED? | DAILY SCORE |
|-----|---------|----------------|-------------|
| MONDAY | | | ☆ ☆ ☆ ☆ ☆ |
| TUESDAY | | | ☆ ☆ ☆ ☆ ☆ |
| WEDNESDAY | | | ☆ ☆ ☆ ☆ ☆ |
| THURSDAY | | | ☆ ☆ ☆ ☆ ☆ |
| FRIDAY | | | ☆ ☆ ☆ ☆ ☆ |
| SATURDAY | | | ☆ ☆ ☆ ☆ ☆ |
| SUNDAY | | | ☆ ☆ ☆ ☆ ☆ |

# Mood Tracker

| MONTH | | | | | WEEK | | | |
|---|---|---|---|---|---|---|---|---|

| | MONDAY | TUESDAY | WEDNESDAY | THURSDAY | FRIDAY | SATURDAY | SUNDAY |
|---|---|---|---|---|---|---|---|
| **HAPPY** | | | | | | | |
| **NEUTRAL** | | | | | | | |
| **SAD** | | | | | | | |

| DAY | EMOTION | WHAT HAPPENED? | DAILY SCORE |
|---|---|---|---|
| MONDAY | | | ☆ ☆ ☆ ☆ ☆ |
| TUESDAY | | | ☆ ☆ ☆ ☆ ☆ |
| WEDNESDAY | | | ☆ ☆ ☆ ☆ ☆ |
| THURSDAY | | | ☆ ☆ ☆ ☆ ☆ |
| FRIDAY | | | ☆ ☆ ☆ ☆ ☆ |
| SATURDAY | | | ☆ ☆ ☆ ☆ ☆ |
| SUNDAY | | | ☆ ☆ ☆ ☆ ☆ |

# Mood Tracker

| MONTH | | | | | | | WEEK | | |
|---|---|---|---|---|---|---|---|---|---|

| | | | | | | | | | |
|---|---|---|---|---|---|---|---|---|---|
| HAPPY | | | | | | | | | |
| NEUTRAL | | | | | | | | | |
| SAD | | | | | | | | | |
| | MONDAY | TUESDAY | WEDNESDAY | THURSDAY | FRIDAY | SATURDAY | SUNDAY | | |

| DAY | EMOTION | WHAT HAPPENED? | DAILY SCORE |
|---|---|---|---|
| MONDAY | | | ☆ ☆ ☆ ☆ ☆ |
| TUESDAY | | | ☆ ☆ ☆ ☆ ☆ |
| WEDNESDAY | | | ☆ ☆ ☆ ☆ ☆ |
| THURSDAY | | | ☆ ☆ ☆ ☆ ☆ |
| FRIDAY | | | ☆ ☆ ☆ ☆ ☆ |
| SATURDAY | | | ☆ ☆ ☆ ☆ ☆ |
| SUNDAY | | | ☆ ☆ ☆ ☆ ☆ |

# Mood Tracker

| MONTH | | | | | | | WEEK | | | |
|-------|---|---|---|---|---|---|------|---|---|---|

| | | | | | | | | | | |
|-------|---|---|---|---|---|---|---|---|---|---|
| HAPPY | | | | | | | | | | |
| NEUTRAL | | | | | | | | | | |
| SAD | | | | | | | | | | |
| | MONDAY | | TUESDAY | | WEDNESDAY | | THURSDAY | | FRIDAY | SATURDAY | SUNDAY |

| DAY | EMOTION | WHAT HAPPENED? | DAILY SCORE |
|-----|---------|----------------|-------------|
| MONDAY | | | ☆ ☆ ☆ ☆ ☆ |
| TUESDAY | | | ☆ ☆ ☆ ☆ ☆ |
| WEDNESDAY | | | ☆ ☆ ☆ ☆ ☆ |
| THURSDAY | | | ☆ ☆ ☆ ☆ ☆ |
| FRIDAY | | | ☆ ☆ ☆ ☆ ☆ |
| SATURDAY | | | ☆ ☆ ☆ ☆ ☆ |
| SUNDAY | | | ☆ ☆ ☆ ☆ ☆ |

# Mood Tracker

| MONTH | | | | | | WEEK | | |
|---|---|---|---|---|---|---|---|---|

| | MONDAY | TUESDAY | WEDNESDAY | THURSDAY | FRIDAY | SATURDAY | SUNDAY |
|---|---|---|---|---|---|---|---|
| **HAPPY** | | | | | | | |
| **NEUTRAL** | | | | | | | |
| **SAD** | | | | | | | |

| DAY | EMOTION | WHAT HAPPENED? | DAILY SCORE |
|---|---|---|---|
| MONDAY | | | ☆ ☆ ☆ ☆ ☆ |
| TUESDAY | | | ☆ ☆ ☆ ☆ ☆ |
| WEDNESDAY | | | ☆ ☆ ☆ ☆ ☆ |
| THURSDAY | | | ☆ ☆ ☆ ☆ ☆ |
| FRIDAY | | | ☆ ☆ ☆ ☆ ☆ |
| SATURDAY | | | ☆ ☆ ☆ ☆ ☆ |
| SUNDAY | | | ☆ ☆ ☆ ☆ ☆ |

# Mood Tracker

| MONTH | | | | | | | | WEEK | | | |

| | | | | | | | | | | | |
|---|---|---|---|---|---|---|---|---|---|---|---|
| **HAPPY** | | | | | | | | | | | |
| **NEUTRAL** | | | | | | | | | | | |
| **SAD** | | | | | | | | | | | |
| | MONDAY | | TUESDAY | | WEDNESDAY | | THURSDAY | | FRIDAY | | SATURDAY | | SUNDAY |

| DAY | EMOTION | WHAT HAPPENED? | DAILY SCORE |
|---|---|---|---|
| MONDAY | | | ☆ ☆ ☆ ☆ ☆ |
| TUESDAY | | | ☆ ☆ ☆ ☆ ☆ |
| WEDNESDAY | | | ☆ ☆ ☆ ☆ ☆ |
| THURSDAY | | | ☆ ☆ ☆ ☆ ☆ |
| FRIDAY | | | ☆ ☆ ☆ ☆ ☆ |
| SATURDAY | | | ☆ ☆ ☆ ☆ ☆ |
| SUNDAY | | | ☆ ☆ ☆ ☆ ☆ |

# Mood Tracker

| MONTH | | | | | | | WEEK | | |
|---|---|---|---|---|---|---|---|---|---|

| | MONDAY | TUESDAY | WEDNESDAY | THURSDAY | FRIDAY | SATURDAY | SUNDAY |
|---|---|---|---|---|---|---|---|
| HAPPY | | | | | | | |
| NEUTRAL | | | | | | | |
| SAD | | | | | | | |

| DAY | EMOTION | WHAT HAPPENED? | DAILY SCORE |
|---|---|---|---|
| MONDAY | | | ☆ ☆ ☆ ☆ ☆ |
| TUESDAY | | | ☆ ☆ ☆ ☆ ☆ |
| WEDNESDAY | | | ☆ ☆ ☆ ☆ ☆ |
| THURSDAY | | | ☆ ☆ ☆ ☆ ★ |
| FRIDAY | | | ☆ ☆ ☆ ☆ ☆ |
| SATURDAY | | | ☆ ☆ ☆ ☆ ☆ |
| SUNDAY | | | ☆ ☆ ☆ ☆ ☆ |

# Mood Tracker

| MONTH | | | WEEK | |
|---|---|---|---|---|

| | MONDAY | TUESDAY | WEDNESDAY | THURSDAY | FRIDAY | SATURDAY | SUNDAY |
|---|---|---|---|---|---|---|---|
| HAPPY | | | | | | | |
| NEUTRAL | | | | | | | |
| SAD | | | | | | | |

| DAY | EMOTION | WHAT HAPPENED? | DAILY SCORE |
|---|---|---|---|
| MONDAY | | | ☆ ☆ ☆ ☆ ☆ |
| TUESDAY | | | ☆ ☆ ☆ ☆ ☆ |
| WEDNESDAY | | | ☆ ☆ ☆ ☆ ☆ |
| THURSDAY | | | ☆ ☆ ☆ ☆ ☆ |
| FRIDAY | | | ☆ ☆ ☆ ☆ ☆ |
| SATURDAY | | | ☆ ☆ ☆ ☆ ☆ |
| SUNDAY | | | ☆ ☆ ☆ ☆ ☆ |

# Mood Tracker

| MONTH | | | | | WEEK | | | |
|---|---|---|---|---|---|---|---|---|

| | | | | | | | |
|---|---|---|---|---|---|---|---|
| **HAPPY** | | | | | | | |
| **NEUTRAL** | | | | | | | |
| **SAD** | | | | | | | |
| | MONDAY | TUESDAY | WEDNESDAY | THURSDAY | FRIDAY | SATURDAY | SUNDAY |

| DAY | EMOTION | WHAT HAPPENED? | DAILY SCORE |
|---|---|---|---|
| MONDAY | | | ☆ ☆ ☆ ☆ ☆ |
| TUESDAY | | | ☆ ☆ ☆ ☆ ☆ |
| WEDNESDAY | | | ☆ ☆ ☆ ☆ ☆ |
| THURSDAY | | | ☆ ☆ ☆ ☆ ☆ |
| FRIDAY | | | ☆ ☆ ☆ ☆ ☆ |
| SATURDAY | | | ☆ ☆ ☆ ☆ ☆ |
| SUNDAY | | | ☆ ☆ ☆ ☆ ☆ |

# Mood Tracker

| MONTH | | | | | | | WEEK | | |
|---|---|---|---|---|---|---|---|---|---|

| | MONDAY | TUESDAY | WEDNESDAY | THURSDAY | FRIDAY | SATURDAY | SUNDAY |
|---|---|---|---|---|---|---|---|
| **HAPPY** | | | | | | | |
| **NEUTRAL** | | | | | | | |
| **SAD** | | | | | | | |

| DAY | EMOTION | WHAT HAPPENED? | DAILY SCORE |
|---|---|---|---|
| MONDAY | | | ☆ ☆ ☆ ☆ ☆ |
| TUESDAY | | | ☆ ☆ ☆ ☆ ☆ |
| WEDNESDAY | | | ☆ ☆ ☆ ☆ ☆ |
| THURSDAY | | | ☆ ☆ ☆ ☆ ☆ |
| FRIDAY | | | ☆ ☆ ☆ ☆ ☆ |
| SATURDAY | | | ☆ ☆ ☆ ☆ ☆ |
| SUNDAY | | | ☆ ☆ ☆ ☆ ☆ |

# Mood Tracker

| MONTH | | WEEK | |
|---|---|---|---|

| | MONDAY | TUESDAY | WEDNESDAY | THURSDAY | FRIDAY | SATURDAY | SUNDAY |
|---|---|---|---|---|---|---|---|
| HAPPY | | | | | | | |
| NEUTRAL | | | | | | | |
| SAD | | | | | | | |

| DAY | EMOTION | WHAT HAPPENED? | DAILY SCORE |
|---|---|---|---|
| MONDAY | | | ☆ ☆ ☆ ☆ ☆ |
| TUESDAY | | | ☆ ☆ ☆ ☆ ☆ |
| WEDNESDAY | | | ☆ ☆ ☆ ☆ ☆ |
| THURSDAY | | | ☆ ☆ ☆ ☆ ☆ |
| FRIDAY | | | ☆ ☆ ☆ ☆ ☆ |
| SATURDAY | | | ☆ ☆ ☆ ☆ ☆ |
| SUNDAY | | | ☆ ☆ ☆ ☆ ☆ |

# Mood Tracker

| MONTH | | | | | | | | WEEK | |
|---|---|---|---|---|---|---|---|---|---|

| | MONDAY | TUESDAY | WEDNESDAY | THURSDAY | FRIDAY | SATURDAY | SUNDAY |
|---|---|---|---|---|---|---|---|
| HAPPY | | | | | | | |
| NEUTRAL | | | | | | | |
| SAD | | | | | | | |

| DAY | EMOTION | WHAT HAPPENED? | DAILY SCORE |
|---|---|---|---|
| MONDAY | | | ☆ ☆ ☆ ☆ ☆ |
| TUESDAY | | | ☆ ☆ ☆ ☆ ☆ |
| WEDNESDAY | | | ☆ ☆ ☆ ☆ ☆ |
| THURSDAY | | | ☆ ☆ ☆ ☆ ☆ |
| FRIDAY | | | ☆ ☆ ☆ ☆ ☆ |
| SATURDAY | | | ☆ ☆ ☆ ☆ ☆ |
| SUNDAY | | | ☆ ☆ ☆ ☆ ☆ |

# Mood Tracker

| MONTH | | | | | | WEEK | | | |
|---|---|---|---|---|---|---|---|---|---|

| | MONDAY | TUESDAY | WEDNESDAY | THURSDAY | FRIDAY | SATURDAY | SUNDAY |
|---|---|---|---|---|---|---|---|
| HAPPY | | | | | | | |
| NEUTRAL | | | | | | | |
| SAD | | | | | | | |

| DAY | EMOTION | WHAT HAPPENED? | DAILY SCORE |
|---|---|---|---|
| MONDAY | | | ☆ ☆ ☆ ☆ ☆ |
| TUESDAY | | | ☆ ☆ ☆ ☆ ☆ |
| WEDNESDAY | | | ☆ ☆ ☆ ☆ ☆ |
| THURSDAY | | | ☆ ☆ ☆ ☆ ☆ |
| FRIDAY | | | ☆ ☆ ☆ ☆ ☆ |
| SATURDAY | | | ☆ ☆ ☆ ☆ ☆ |
| SUNDAY | | | ☆ ☆ ☆ ☆ ☆ |

# Mood Tracker

| MONTH | | | | | | WEEK | | | |
|---|---|---|---|---|---|---|---|---|---|

| | MONDAY | TUESDAY | WEDNESDAY | THURSDAY | FRIDAY | SATURDAY | SUNDAY |
|---|---|---|---|---|---|---|---|
| HAPPY | | | | | | | |
| NEUTRAL | | | | | | | |
| SAD | | | | | | | |

| DAY | EMOTION | WHAT HAPPENED? | DAILY SCORE |
|---|---|---|---|
| MONDAY | | | ☆ ☆ ☆ ☆ ☆ |
| TUESDAY | | | ☆ ☆ ☆ ☆ ☆ |
| WEDNESDAY | | | ☆ ☆ ☆ ☆ ☆ |
| THURSDAY | | | ☆ ☆ ☆ ☆ ☆ |
| FRIDAY | | | ☆ ☆ ☆ ☆ ☆ |
| SATURDAY | | | ☆ ☆ ☆ ☆ ☆ |
| SUNDAY | | | ☆ ☆ ☆ ☆ ☆ |

# Mood Tracker

| MONTH | | | | | WEEK | | | |
|-------|--|--|--|--|------|--|--|--|

| | | | | | | | | |
|---|---|---|---|---|---|---|---|---|
| HAPPY | | | | | | | | |
| NEUTRAL | | | | | | | | |
| SAD | | | | | | | | |
| | MONDAY | TUESDAY | WEDNESDAY | THURSDAY | FRIDAY | SATURDAY | SUNDAY | |

| DAY | EMOTION | WHAT HAPPENED? | DAILY SCORE |
|-----|---------|----------------|-------------|
| MONDAY | | | ☆ ☆ ☆ ☆ ☆ |
| TUESDAY | | | ☆ ☆ ☆ ☆ ☆ |
| WEDNESDAY | | | ☆ ☆ ☆ ☆ ☆ |
| THURSDAY | | | ☆ ☆ ☆ ☆ ☆ |
| FRIDAY | | | ☆ ☆ ☆ ☆ ☆ |
| SATURDAY | | | ☆ ☆ ☆ ☆ ☆ |
| SUNDAY | | | ☆ ☆ ☆ ☆ ☆ |

# Mood Tracker

| MONTH | | | | | WEEK | | |
|---|---|---|---|---|---|---|---|

| | MONDAY | TUESDAY | WEDNESDAY | THURSDAY | FRIDAY | SATURDAY | SUNDAY |
|---|---|---|---|---|---|---|---|
| HAPPY | | | | | | | |
| NEUTRAL | | | | | | | |
| SAD | | | | | | | |

| DAY | EMOTION | WHAT HAPPENED? | DAILY SCORE |
|---|---|---|---|
| MONDAY | | | ☆ ☆ ☆ ☆ ☆ |
| TUESDAY | | | ☆ ☆ ☆ ☆ ☆ |
| WEDNESDAY | | | ☆ ☆ ☆ ☆ ☆ |
| THURSDAY | | | ☆ ☆ ☆ ☆ ☆ |
| FRIDAY | | | ☆ ☆ ☆ ☆ ☆ |
| SATURDAY | | | ☆ ☆ ☆ ☆ ☆ |
| SUNDAY | | | ☆ ☆ ☆ ☆ ☆ |

# Mood Tracker

| MONTH | | | | WEEK | | | |
|---|---|---|---|---|---|---|---|

| | MONDAY | TUESDAY | WEDNESDAY | THURSDAY | FRIDAY | SATURDAY | SUNDAY |
|---|---|---|---|---|---|---|---|
| HAPPY | | | | | | | |
| NEUTRAL | | | | | | | |
| SAD | | | | | | | |

| DAY | EMOTION | WHAT HAPPENED? | DAILY SCORE |
|---|---|---|---|
| MONDAY | | | ☆ ☆ ☆ ☆ ☆ |
| TUESDAY | | | ☆ ☆ ☆ ☆ ☆ |
| WEDNESDAY | | | ☆ ☆ ☆ ☆ ☆ |
| THURSDAY | | | ☆ ☆ ★ ☆ ☆ |
| FRIDAY | | | ☆ ☆ ☆ ☆ ☆ |
| SATURDAY | | | ☆ ☆ ☆ ☆ ☆ |
| SUNDAY | | | ☆ ☆ ☆ ☆ ☆ |

# Mood Tracker

| MONTH | | | | | | WEEK | | |
|---|---|---|---|---|---|---|---|---|

| | | | | | | | | |
|---|---|---|---|---|---|---|---|---|
| **HAPPY** | | | | | | | | |
| **NEUTRAL** | | | | | | | | |
| **SAD** | | | | | | | | |
| | MONDAY | TUESDAY | WEDNESDAY | THURSDAY | FRIDAY | SATURDAY | SUNDAY | |

| DAY | EMOTION | WHAT HAPPENED? | DAILY SCORE |
|---|---|---|---|
| MONDAY | | | ☆ ☆ ☆ ☆ ☆ |
| TUESDAY | | | ☆ ☆ ☆ ☆ ☆ |
| WEDNESDAY | | | ☆ ☆ ☆ ☆ ☆ |
| THURSDAY | | | ☆ ☆ ☆ ☆ ☆ |
| FRIDAY | | | ☆ ☆ ☆ ☆ ☆ |
| SATURDAY | | | ☆ ☆ ☆ ☆ ☆ |
| SUNDAY | | | ☆ ☆ ☆ ☆ ☆ |

# Mood Tracker

| MONTH | | | | WEEK | | | |
|-------|--|--|--|------|--|--|--|

|  | MONDAY | TUESDAY | WEDNESDAY | THURSDAY | FRIDAY | SATURDAY | SUNDAY |
|------|--------|---------|-----------|----------|--------|----------|--------|
| HAPPY | | | | | | | |
| NEUTRAL | | | | | | | |
| SAD | | | | | | | |

| DAY | EMOTION | WHAT HAPPENED? | DAILY SCORE |
|-----|---------|----------------|-------------|
| MONDAY | | | ☆ ☆ ☆ ☆ ☆ |
| TUESDAY | | | ☆ ☆ ☆ ☆ ☆ |
| WEDNESDAY | | | ☆ ☆ ☆ ☆ ☆ |
| THURSDAY | | | ★ ☆ ☆ ☆ ☆ |
| FRIDAY | | | ☆ ☆ ☆ ☆ ☆ |
| SATURDAY | | | ☆ ☆ ☆ ☆ ☆ |
| SUNDAY | | | ☆ ☆ ☆ ☆ ☆ |

# Mood Tracker

| MONTH | | | | WEEK | | | |
|---|---|---|---|---|---|---|---|

|  | MONDAY | TUESDAY | WEDNESDAY | THURSDAY | FRIDAY | SATURDAY | SUNDAY |
|---|---|---|---|---|---|---|---|
| HAPPY | | | | | | | |
| NEUTRAL | | | | | | | |
| SAD | | | | | | | |

| DAY | EMOTION | WHAT HAPPENED? | DAILY SCORE |
|---|---|---|---|
| MONDAY | | | ☆ ☆ ☆ ☆ ☆ |
| TUESDAY | | | ☆ ☆ ☆ ☆ ☆ |
| WEDNESDAY | | | ☆ ☆ ☆ ☆ ☆ |
| THURSDAY | | | ☆ ☆ ☆ ☆ ☆ |
| FRIDAY | | | ☆ ☆ ☆ ☆ ☆ |
| SATURDAY | | | ☆ ☆ ☆ ☆ ☆ |
| SUNDAY | | | ☆ ☆ ☆ ☆ ☆ |

# Mood Tracker

| MONTH | | | | | | | WEEK | | |
|---|---|---|---|---|---|---|---|---|---|

| | MONDAY | TUESDAY | WEDNESDAY | THURSDAY | FRIDAY | SATURDAY | SUNDAY |
|---|---|---|---|---|---|---|---|
| HAPPY | | | | | | | |
| NEUTRAL | | | | | | | |
| SAD | | | | | | | |

| DAY | EMOTION | WHAT HAPPENED? | DAILY SCORE |
|---|---|---|---|
| MONDAY | | | ☆ ☆ ☆ ☆ ☆ |
| TUESDAY | | | ☆ ☆ ☆ ☆ ☆ |
| WEDNESDAY | | | ☆ ☆ ☆ ☆ ☆ |
| THURSDAY | | | ☆ ☆ ☆ ☆ ☆ |
| FRIDAY | | | ☆ ☆ ☆ ☆ ☆ |
| SATURDAY | | | ☆ ☆ ☆ ☆ ☆ |
| SUNDAY | | | ☆ ☆ ☆ ☆ ☆ |

# Mood Tracker

| MONTH | | WEEK | |
|---|---|---|---|

| | | | | | | | |
|---|---|---|---|---|---|---|---|
| **HAPPY** | | | | | | | |
| **NEUTRAL** | | | | | | | |
| **SAD** | | | | | | | |
| | MONDAY | TUESDAY | WEDNESDAY | THURSDAY | FRIDAY | SATURDAY | SUNDAY |

| DAY | EMOTION | WHAT HAPPENED? | DAILY SCORE |
|---|---|---|---|
| MONDAY | | | ★ ★ ★ ★ ☆ |
| TUESDAY | | | ★ ★ ★ ★ ☆ |
| WEDNESDAY | | | ★ ★ ★ ★ ☆ |
| THURSDAY | | | ★ ★ ★ ★ ☆ |
| FRIDAY | | | ★ ★ ★ ★ ☆ |
| SATURDAY | | | ★ ★ ★ ★ ☆ |
| SUNDAY | | | ★ ★ ★ ★ ☆ |

# Mood Tracker

| MONTH | | WEEK | |
|---|---|---|---|

| | MONDAY | TUESDAY | WEDNESDAY | THURSDAY | FRIDAY | SATURDAY | SUNDAY |
|---|---|---|---|---|---|---|---|
| HAPPY | | | | | | | |
| NEUTRAL | | | | | | | |
| SAD | | | | | | | |

| DAY | EMOTION | WHAT HAPPENED? | DAILY SCORE |
|---|---|---|---|
| MONDAY | | | ☆ ☆ ☆ ☆ ☆ |
| TUESDAY | | | ☆ ☆ ☆ ☆ ☆ |
| WEDNESDAY | | | ☆ ☆ ☆ ☆ ☆ |
| THURSDAY | | | ☆ ☆ ☆ ☆ ☆ |
| FRIDAY | | | ☆ ☆ ☆ ☆ ☆ |
| SATURDAY | | | ☆ ☆ ☆ ☆ ☆ |
| SUNDAY | | | ☆ ☆ ☆ ☆ ☆ |

# Mood Tracker

| MONTH | | | | | | WEEK | | |
|---|---|---|---|---|---|---|---|---|

| | MONDAY | TUESDAY | WEDNESDAY | THURSDAY | FRIDAY | SATURDAY | SUNDAY |
|---|---|---|---|---|---|---|---|
| **HAPPY** | | | | | | | |
| **NEUTRAL** | | | | | | | |
| **SAD** | | | | | | | |

| DAY | EMOTION | WHAT HAPPENED? | DAILY SCORE |
|---|---|---|---|
| MONDAY | | | ☆ ☆ ☆ ☆ ☆ |
| TUESDAY | | | ☆ ☆ ☆ ☆ ☆ |
| WEDNESDAY | | | ☆ ☆ ☆ ☆ ☆ |
| THURSDAY | | | ☆ ☆ ☆ ☆ ☆ |
| FRIDAY | | | ☆ ☆ ☆ ☆ ☆ |
| SATURDAY | | | ☆ ☆ ☆ ☆ ☆ |
| SUNDAY | | | ☆ ☆ ☆ ☆ ☆ |

# Mood Tracker

| MONTH | | | | WEEK | | | |
|---|---|---|---|---|---|---|---|

| | MONDAY | TUESDAY | WEDNESDAY | THURSDAY | FRIDAY | SATURDAY | SUNDAY |
|---|---|---|---|---|---|---|---|
| HAPPY | | | | | | | |
| NEUTRAL | | | | | | | |
| SAD | | | | | | | |

| DAY | EMOTION | WHAT HAPPENED? | DAILY SCORE |
|---|---|---|---|
| MONDAY | | | ☆ ☆ ☆ ☆ ☆ |
| TUESDAY | | | ☆ ☆ ☆ ☆ ☆ |
| WEDNESDAY | | | ☆ ☆ ☆ ☆ ☆ |
| THURSDAY | | | ☆ ☆ ☆ ☆ ☆ |
| FRIDAY | | | ☆ ☆ ☆ ☆ ☆ |
| SATURDAY | | | ☆ ☆ ☆ ☆ ☆ |
| SUNDAY | | | ☆ ☆ ☆ ☆ ☆ |

# Mood Tracker

| MONTH | | | | | | WEEK | | | |
|---|---|---|---|---|---|---|---|---|---|

| | MONDAY | TUESDAY | WEDNESDAY | THURSDAY | FRIDAY | SATURDAY | SUNDAY |
|---|---|---|---|---|---|---|---|
| HAPPY | | | | | | | |
| NEUTRAL | | | | | | | |
| SAD | | | | | | | |

| DAY | EMOTION | WHAT HAPPENED? | DAILY SCORE |
|---|---|---|---|
| MONDAY | | | ☆ ☆ ☆ ☆ ☆ |
| TUESDAY | | | ☆ ☆ ☆ ☆ ☆ |
| WEDNESDAY | | | ☆ ☆ ☆ ☆ ☆ |
| THURSDAY | | | ☆ ☆ ☆ ☆ ☆ |
| FRIDAY | | | ☆ ☆ ☆ ☆ ☆ |
| SATURDAY | | | ☆ ☆ ☆ ☆ ☆ |
| SUNDAY | | | ☆ ☆ ☆ ☆ ☆ |

# Mood Tracker

| MONTH | | WEEK | |
|---|---|---|---|

| | MONDAY | TUESDAY | WEDNESDAY | THURSDAY | FRIDAY | SATURDAY | SUNDAY |
|---|---|---|---|---|---|---|---|
| **HAPPY** | | | | | | | |
| **NEUTRAL** | | | | | | | |
| **SAD** | | | | | | | |

| DAY | EMOTION | WHAT HAPPENED? | DAILY SCORE |
|---|---|---|---|
| MONDAY | | | ☆ ☆ ☆ ☆ ☆ |
| TUESDAY | | | ☆ ☆ ☆ ☆ ☆ |
| WEDNESDAY | | | ☆ ☆ ☆ ☆ ☆ |
| THURSDAY | | | ☆ ☆ ☆ ☆ ☆ |
| FRIDAY | | | ☆ ☆ ☆ ☆ ☆ |
| SATURDAY | | | ☆ ☆ ☆ ☆ ☆ |
| SUNDAY | | | ☆ ☆ ☆ ☆ ☆ |

# Mood Tracker

| MONTH | | WEEK | |
|---|---|---|---|

| | MONDAY | TUESDAY | WEDNESDAY | THURSDAY | FRIDAY | SATURDAY | SUNDAY |
|---|---|---|---|---|---|---|---|
| HAPPY | | | | | | | |
| NEUTRAL | | | | | | | |
| SAD | | | | | | | |

| DAY | EMOTION | WHAT HAPPENED? | DAILY SCORE |
|---|---|---|---|
| MONDAY | | | ☆ ☆ ☆ ☆ ☆ |
| TUESDAY | | | ☆ ☆ ☆ ☆ ☆ |
| WEDNESDAY | | | ☆ ☆ ☆ ☆ ☆ |
| THURSDAY | | | ☆ ☆ ☆ ☆ ☆ |
| FRIDAY | | | ☆ ☆ ☆ ☆ ☆ |
| SATURDAY | | | ☆ ☆ ☆ ☆ ☆ |
| SUNDAY | | | ☆ ☆ ☆ ☆ ☆ |

# Mood Tracker

| MONTH | | | | | | WEEK | |
|---|---|---|---|---|---|---|---|

| | MONDAY | TUESDAY | WEDNESDAY | THURSDAY | FRIDAY | SATURDAY | SUNDAY |
|---|---|---|---|---|---|---|---|
| HAPPY | | | | | | | |
| NEUTRAL | | | | | | | |
| SAD | | | | | | | |

| DAY | EMOTION | WHAT HAPPENED? | DAILY SCORE |
|---|---|---|---|
| MONDAY | | | ☆ ☆ ☆ ☆ ☆ |
| TUESDAY | | | ☆ ☆ ☆ ☆ ☆ |
| WEDNESDAY | | | ☆ ☆ ☆ ☆ ☆ |
| THURSDAY | | | ☆ ☆ ☆ ☆ ☆ |
| FRIDAY | | | ☆ ☆ ☆ ☆ ☆ |
| SATURDAY | | | ☆ ☆ ☆ ☆ ☆ |
| SUNDAY | | | ☆ ☆ ☆ ☆ ☆ |

# Mood Tracker

| MONTH | | | | | WEEK | | |
|---|---|---|---|---|---|---|---|

| | MONDAY | TUESDAY | WEDNESDAY | THURSDAY | FRIDAY | SATURDAY | SUNDAY |
|---|---|---|---|---|---|---|---|
| **HAPPY** | | | | | | | |
| **NEUTRAL** | | | | | | | |
| **SAD** | | | | | | | |

| DAY | EMOTION | WHAT HAPPENED? | DAILY SCORE |
|---|---|---|---|
| MONDAY | | | ☆ ☆ ☆ ☆ ☆ |
| TUESDAY | | | ☆ ☆ ☆ ☆ ☆ |
| WEDNESDAY | | | ☆ ☆ ☆ ☆ ☆ |
| THURSDAY | | | ☆ ☆ ☆ ☆ ☆ |
| FRIDAY | | | ☆ ☆ ☆ ☆ ☆ |
| SATURDAY | | | ☆ ☆ ☆ ☆ ☆ |
| SUNDAY | | | ☆ ☆ ☆ ☆ ☆ |

# Mood Tracker

| MONTH | | WEEK | |
|---|---|---|---|

| | | | | | | | |
|---|---|---|---|---|---|---|---|
| HAPPY | | | | | | | |
| NEUTRAL | | | | | | | |
| SAD | | | | | | | |
| | MONDAY | TUESDAY | WEDNESDAY | THURSDAY | FRIDAY | SATURDAY | SUNDAY |

| DAY | EMOTION | WHAT HAPPENED? | DAILY SCORE |
|---|---|---|---|
| MONDAY | | | ☆ ☆ ☆ ☆ ☆ |
| TUESDAY | | | ☆ ☆ ☆ ☆ ☆ |
| WEDNESDAY | | | ☆ ☆ ☆ ☆ ☆ |
| THURSDAY | | | ★ ☆ ☆ ☆ ☆ |
| FRIDAY | | | ☆ ☆ ☆ ☆ ☆ |
| SATURDAY | | | ☆ ☆ ☆ ☆ ☆ |
| SUNDAY | | | ☆ ☆ ☆ ☆ ☆ |

# Mood Tracker

| MONTH | | | WEEK | | |
|-------|---|---|------|---|---|

|  | MONDAY | TUESDAY | WEDNESDAY | THURSDAY | FRIDAY | SATURDAY | SUNDAY |
|--------|--------|---------|-----------|----------|--------|----------|--------|
| HAPPY | | | | | | | |
| NEUTRAL | | | | | | | |
| SAD | | | | | | | |

| DAY | EMOTION | WHAT HAPPENED? | DAILY SCORE |
|-----|---------|----------------|-------------|
| MONDAY | | | ☆ ☆ ☆ ☆ ☆ |
| TUESDAY | | | ☆ ☆ ☆ ☆ ☆ |
| WEDNESDAY | | | ☆ ☆ ☆ ☆ ☆ |
| THURSDAY | | | ☆ ☆ ☆ ☆ ☆ |
| FRIDAY | | | ☆ ☆ ☆ ☆ ☆ |
| SATURDAY | | | ☆ ☆ ☆ ☆ ☆ |
| SUNDAY | | | ☆ ☆ ☆ ☆ ☆ |

# Mood Tracker

| MONTH | | WEEK | |
|---|---|---|---|

| | | | | | | | |
|---|---|---|---|---|---|---|---|
| **HAPPY** | | | | | | | |
| **NEUTRAL** | | | | | | | |
| **SAD** | | | | | | | |
| | MONDAY | TUESDAY | WEDNESDAY | THURSDAY | FRIDAY | SATURDAY | SUNDAY |

| DAY | EMOTION | WHAT HAPPENED? | DAILY SCORE |
|---|---|---|---|
| MONDAY | | | ☆ ☆ ☆ ☆ ☆ |
| TUESDAY | | | ☆ ☆ ☆ ☆ ☆ |
| WEDNESDAY | | | ☆ ☆ ☆ ☆ ☆ |
| THURSDAY | | | ☆ ☆ ☆ ☆ ☆ |
| FRIDAY | | | ☆ ☆ ☆ ☆ ☆ |
| SATURDAY | | | ☆ ☆ ☆ ☆ ☆ |
| SUNDAY | | | ☆ ☆ ☆ ☆ ☆ |

# Mood Tracker

| MONTH | | | | | WEEK | | |
|---|---|---|---|---|---|---|---|

| | MONDAY | TUESDAY | WEDNESDAY | THURSDAY | FRIDAY | SATURDAY | SUNDAY |
|---|---|---|---|---|---|---|---|
| HAPPY | | | | | | | |
| NEUTRAL | | | | | | | |
| SAD | | | | | | | |

| DAY | EMOTION | WHAT HAPPENED? | DAILY SCORE |
|---|---|---|---|
| MONDAY | | | ☆ ☆ ☆ ☆ ☆ |
| TUESDAY | | | ☆ ☆ ☆ ☆ ☆ |
| WEDNESDAY | | | ☆ ☆ ☆ ☆ ☆ |
| THURSDAY | | | ☆ ☆ ☆ ☆ ☆ |
| FRIDAY | | | ☆ ☆ ☆ ☆ ☆ |
| SATURDAY | | | ☆ ☆ ☆ ☆ ☆ |
| SUNDAY | | | ☆ ☆ ☆ ☆ ☆ |

# Mood Tracker

| MONTH | | WEEK | |
|---|---|---|---|

| | | | | | | | |
|---|---|---|---|---|---|---|---|
| HAPPY | | | | | | | |
| NEUTRAL | | | | | | | |
| SAD | | | | | | | |
| | MONDAY | TUESDAY | WEDNESDAY | THURSDAY | FRIDAY | SATURDAY | SUNDAY |

| DAY | EMOTION | WHAT HAPPENED? | DAILY SCORE |
|---|---|---|---|
| MONDAY | | | ☆ ☆ ☆ ☆ ☆ |
| TUESDAY | | | ☆ ☆ ☆ ☆ ☆ |
| WEDNESDAY | | | ☆ ☆ ☆ ☆ ☆ |
| THURSDAY | | | ☆ ☆ ☆ ☆ ☆ |
| FRIDAY | | | ☆ ☆ ☆ ☆ ☆ |
| SATURDAY | | | ☆ ☆ ☆ ☆ ☆ |
| SUNDAY | | | ☆ ☆ ☆ ☆ ☆ |

# Mood Tracker

| MONTH | | | | WEEK | | |
|---|---|---|---|---|---|---|

| | MONDAY | TUESDAY | WEDNESDAY | THURSDAY | FRIDAY | SATURDAY | SUNDAY |
|---|---|---|---|---|---|---|---|
| HAPPY | | | | | | | |
| NEUTRAL | | | | | | | |
| SAD | | | | | | | |

| DAY | EMOTION | WHAT HAPPENED? | DAILY SCORE |
|---|---|---|---|
| MONDAY | | | ☆ ☆ ☆ ☆ ☆ |
| TUESDAY | | | ☆ ☆ ☆ ☆ ☆ |
| WEDNESDAY | | | ☆ ☆ ☆ ☆ ☆ |
| THURSDAY | | | ☆ ☆ ☆ ☆ ☆ |
| FRIDAY | | | ☆ ☆ ☆ ☆ ☆ |
| SATURDAY | | | ☆ ☆ ☆ ☆ ☆ |
| SUNDAY | | | ☆ ☆ ☆ ☆ ☆ |

# Mood Tracker

| MONTH | | WEEK | |
|---|---|---|---|

| | MONDAY | TUESDAY | WEDNESDAY | THURSDAY | FRIDAY | SATURDAY | SUNDAY |
|---|---|---|---|---|---|---|---|
| HAPPY | | | | | | | |
| NEUTRAL | | | | | | | |
| SAD | | | | | | | |

| DAY | EMOTION | WHAT HAPPENED? | DAILY SCORE |
|---|---|---|---|
| MONDAY | | | ☆ ☆ ☆ ☆ ☆ |
| TUESDAY | | | ☆ ☆ ☆ ☆ ☆ |
| WEDNESDAY | | | ☆ ☆ ☆ ☆ ☆ |
| THURSDAY | | | ★ ★ ☆ ☆ ☆ |
| FRIDAY | | | ☆ ☆ ☆ ☆ ☆ |
| SATURDAY | | | ☆ ☆ ☆ ☆ ☆ |
| SUNDAY | | | ☆ ☆ ☆ ☆ ☆ |

# Mood Tracker

| MONTH | | | | | | WEEK | | | |
|---|---|---|---|---|---|---|---|---|---|

| | MONDAY | TUESDAY | WEDNESDAY | THURSDAY | FRIDAY | SATURDAY | SUNDAY |
|---|---|---|---|---|---|---|---|
| **HAPPY** | | | | | | | |
| **NEUTRAL** | | | | | | | |
| **SAD** | | | | | | | |

| DAY | EMOTION | WHAT HAPPENED? | DAILY SCORE |
|---|---|---|---|
| MONDAY | | | ☆ ☆ ☆ ☆ ☆ |
| TUESDAY | | | ☆ ☆ ☆ ☆ ☆ |
| WEDNESDAY | | | ☆ ☆ ☆ ☆ ☆ |
| THURSDAY | | | ☆ ☆ ☆ ☆ ☆ |
| FRIDAY | | | ☆ ☆ ☆ ☆ ☆ |
| SATURDAY | | | ☆ ☆ ☆ ☆ ☆ |
| SUNDAY | | | ☆ ☆ ☆ ☆ ☆ |

# Mood Tracker

| MONTH | | | | | | | WEEK | |
|---|---|---|---|---|---|---|---|---|
| HAPPY | | | | | | | | |
| NEUTRAL | | | | | | | | |
| SAD | | | | | | | | |
| | MONDAY | TUESDAY | WEDNESDAY | THURSDAY | FRIDAY | SATURDAY | SUNDAY | |

| DAY | EMOTION | WHAT HAPPENED? | DAILY SCORE |
|---|---|---|---|
| MONDAY | | | ☆ ☆ ☆ ☆ ☆ |
| TUESDAY | | | ☆ ☆ ☆ ☆ ☆ |
| WEDNESDAY | | | ☆ ☆ ☆ ☆ ☆ |
| THURSDAY | | | ☆ ☆ ☆ ☆ ☆ |
| FRIDAY | | | ☆ ☆ ☆ ☆ ☆ |
| SATURDAY | | | ☆ ☆ ☆ ☆ ☆ |
| SUNDAY | | | ☆ ☆ ☆ ☆ ☆ |

# Mood Tracker

| MONTH | | | | | | WEEK | | |
|---|---|---|---|---|---|---|---|---|

| | MONDAY | TUESDAY | WEDNESDAY | THURSDAY | FRIDAY | SATURDAY | SUNDAY |
|---|---|---|---|---|---|---|---|
| **HAPPY** | | | | | | | |
| **NEUTRAL** | | | | | | | |
| **SAD** | | | | | | | |

| DAY | EMOTION | WHAT HAPPENED? | DAILY SCORE |
|---|---|---|---|
| MONDAY | | | ☆ ☆ ☆ ☆ ☆ |
| TUESDAY | | | ☆ ☆ ☆ ☆ ☆ |
| WEDNESDAY | | | ☆ ☆ ☆ ☆ ☆ |
| THURSDAY | | | ☆ ☆ ☆ ☆ ☆ |
| FRIDAY | | | ☆ ☆ ☆ ☆ ☆ |
| SATURDAY | | | ☆ ☆ ☆ ☆ ☆ |
| SUNDAY | | | ☆ ☆ ☆ ☆ ☆ |

# Mood Tracker

| MONTH | | WEEK | |
|---|---|---|---|

| | MONDAY | TUESDAY | WEDNESDAY | THURSDAY | FRIDAY | SATURDAY | SUNDAY |
|---|---|---|---|---|---|---|---|
| HAPPY | | | | | | | |
| NEUTRAL | | | | | | | |
| SAD | | | | | | | |

| DAY | EMOTION | WHAT HAPPENED? | DAILY SCORE |
|---|---|---|---|
| MONDAY | | | ☆ ☆ ☆ ☆ ☆ |
| TUESDAY | | | ☆ ☆ ☆ ☆ ☆ |
| WEDNESDAY | | | ☆ ☆ ☆ ☆ ☆ |
| THURSDAY | | | ☆ ☆ ☆ ☆ ☆ |
| FRIDAY | | | ☆ ☆ ☆ ☆ ☆ |
| SATURDAY | | | ☆ ☆ ☆ ☆ ☆ |
| SUNDAY | | | ☆ ☆ ☆ ☆ ☆ |

# Mood Tracker

| MONTH | | | | | | WEEK | | |
|---|---|---|---|---|---|---|---|---|

| | MONDAY | TUESDAY | WEDNESDAY | THURSDAY | FRIDAY | SATURDAY | SUNDAY |
|---|---|---|---|---|---|---|---|
| HAPPY | | | | | | | |
| NEUTRAL | | | | | | | |
| SAD | | | | | | | |

| DAY | EMOTION | WHAT HAPPENED? | DAILY SCORE |
|---|---|---|---|
| MONDAY | | | ★ ★ ★ ★ ☆ |
| TUESDAY | | | ★ ★ ★ ★ ☆ |
| WEDNESDAY | | | ★ ★ ★ ★ ☆ |
| THURSDAY | | | ★ ★ ★ ★ ☆ |
| FRIDAY | | | ★ ★ ★ ★ ☆ |
| SATURDAY | | | ★ ★ ★ ★ ☆ |
| SUNDAY | | | ★ ★ ★ ★ ☆ |

# Mood Tracker

| MONTH | | | | WEEK | | |
|---|---|---|---|---|---|---|

| | MONDAY | TUESDAY | WEDNESDAY | THURSDAY | FRIDAY | SATURDAY | SUNDAY |
|---|---|---|---|---|---|---|---|
| HAPPY | | | | | | | |
| NEUTRAL | | | | | | | |
| SAD | | | | | | | |

| DAY | EMOTION | WHAT HAPPENED? | DAILY SCORE |
|---|---|---|---|
| MONDAY | | | ☆ ☆ ☆ ☆ ☆ |
| TUESDAY | | | ☆ ☆ ☆ ☆ ☆ |
| WEDNESDAY | | | ☆ ☆ ☆ ☆ ☆ |
| THURSDAY | | | ☆ ☆ ☆ ☆ ☆ |
| FRIDAY | | | ☆ ☆ ☆ ☆ ☆ |
| SATURDAY | | | ☆ ☆ ☆ ☆ ☆ |
| SUNDAY | | | ☆ ☆ ☆ ☆ ☆ |

# Mood Tracker

| MONTH | | | WEEK | | |
|---|---|---|---|---|---|

| | MONDAY | TUESDAY | WEDNESDAY | THURSDAY | FRIDAY | SATURDAY | SUNDAY |
|---|---|---|---|---|---|---|---|
| HAPPY | | | | | | | |
| NEUTRAL | | | | | | | |
| SAD | | | | | | | |

| DAY | EMOTION | WHAT HAPPENED? | DAILY SCORE |
|---|---|---|---|
| MONDAY | | | ☆ ☆ ☆ ☆ ☆ |
| TUESDAY | | | ☆ ☆ ☆ ☆ ☆ |
| WEDNESDAY | | | ☆ ☆ ☆ ☆ ☆ |
| THURSDAY | | | ☆ ☆ ☆ ☆ ☆ |
| FRIDAY | | | ☆ ☆ ☆ ☆ ☆ |
| SATURDAY | | | ☆ ☆ ☆ ☆ ☆ |
| SUNDAY | | | ☆ ☆ ☆ ☆ ☆ |

# Mood Tracker

| MONTH | | | | | WEEK | | |
|---|---|---|---|---|---|---|---|

| | MONDAY | TUESDAY | WEDNESDAY | THURSDAY | FRIDAY | SATURDAY | SUNDAY |
|---|---|---|---|---|---|---|---|
| HAPPY | | | | | | | |
| NEUTRAL | | | | | | | |
| SAD | | | | | | | |

| DAY | EMOTION | WHAT HAPPENED? | DAILY SCORE |
|---|---|---|---|
| MONDAY | | | ☆ ☆ ☆ ☆ ☆ |
| TUESDAY | | | ☆ ☆ ☆ ☆ ☆ |
| WEDNESDAY | | | ☆ ☆ ☆ ☆ ☆ |
| THURSDAY | | | ☆ ☆ ☆ ☆ ☆ |
| FRIDAY | | | ☆ ☆ ☆ ☆ ☆ |
| SATURDAY | | | ☆ ☆ ☆ ☆ ☆ |
| SUNDAY | | | ☆ ☆ ☆ ☆ ☆ |

# Mood Tracker

| MONTH | | | | | | | WEEK | | |
|---|---|---|---|---|---|---|---|---|---|

| | MONDAY | TUESDAY | WEDNESDAY | THURSDAY | FRIDAY | SATURDAY | SUNDAY |
|---|---|---|---|---|---|---|---|
| HAPPY | | | | | | | |
| NEUTRAL | | | | | | | |
| SAD | | | | | | | |

| DAY | EMOTION | WHAT HAPPENED? | DAILY SCORE |
|---|---|---|---|
| MONDAY | | | ☆ ☆ ☆ ☆ ☆ |
| TUESDAY | | | ☆ ☆ ☆ ☆ ☆ |
| WEDNESDAY | | | ☆ ☆ ☆ ☆ ☆ |
| THURSDAY | | | ☆ ☆ ☆ ☆ ☆ |
| FRIDAY | | | ☆ ☆ ☆ ☆ ☆ |
| SATURDAY | | | ☆ ☆ ☆ ☆ ☆ |
| SUNDAY | | | ☆ ☆ ☆ ☆ ☆ |

# Mood Tracker

| MONTH | | | | WEEK | | | |
|---|---|---|---|---|---|---|---|

| | MONDAY | TUESDAY | WEDNESDAY | THURSDAY | FRIDAY | SATURDAY | SUNDAY |
|---|---|---|---|---|---|---|---|
| HAPPY | | | | | | | |
| NEUTRAL | | | | | | | |
| SAD | | | | | | | |

| DAY | EMOTION | WHAT HAPPENED? | DAILY SCORE |
|---|---|---|---|
| MONDAY | | | ☆ ☆ ☆ ☆ ☆ |
| TUESDAY | | | ☆ ☆ ☆ ☆ ☆ |
| WEDNESDAY | | | ☆ ☆ ☆ ☆ ☆ |
| THURSDAY | | | ☆ ☆ ☆ ☆ ☆ |
| FRIDAY | | | ☆ ☆ ☆ ☆ ☆ |
| SATURDAY | | | ☆ ☆ ☆ ☆ ☆ |
| SUNDAY | | | ☆ ☆ ☆ ☆ ☆ |

# Mood Tracker

| MONTH | | | | | | | WEEK | |
|---|---|---|---|---|---|---|---|---|

| | MONDAY | TUESDAY | WEDNESDAY | THURSDAY | FRIDAY | SATURDAY | SUNDAY |
|---|---|---|---|---|---|---|---|
| HAPPY | | | | | | | |
| NEUTRAL | | | | | | | |
| SAD | | | | | | | |

| DAY | EMOTION | WHAT HAPPENED? | DAILY SCORE |
|---|---|---|---|
| MONDAY | | | ☆ ☆ ☆ ☆ ☆ |
| TUESDAY | | | ☆ ☆ ☆ ☆ ☆ |
| WEDNESDAY | | | ☆ ☆ ☆ ☆ ☆ |
| THURSDAY | | | ☆ ☆ ☆ ☆ ☆ |
| FRIDAY | | | ☆ ☆ ☆ ☆ ☆ |
| SATURDAY | | | ☆ ☆ ☆ ☆ ☆ |
| SUNDAY | | | ☆ ☆ ☆ ☆ ☆ |

# Mood Tracker

| MONTH | | WEEK | |
|---|---|---|---|

| | MONDAY | TUESDAY | WEDNESDAY | THURSDAY | FRIDAY | SATURDAY | SUNDAY |
|---|---|---|---|---|---|---|---|
| HAPPY | | | | | | | |
| NEUTRAL | | | | | | | |
| SAD | | | | | | | |

| DAY | EMOTION | WHAT HAPPENED? | DAILY SCORE |
|---|---|---|---|
| MONDAY | | | ☆ ☆ ☆ ☆ ☆ |
| TUESDAY | | | ☆ ☆ ☆ ☆ ☆ |
| WEDNESDAY | | | ☆ ☆ ☆ ☆ ☆ |
| THURSDAY | | | ☆ ☆ ☆ ☆ ☆ |
| FRIDAY | | | ☆ ☆ ☆ ☆ ☆ |
| SATURDAY | | | ☆ ☆ ☆ ☆ ☆ |
| SUNDAY | | | ☆ ☆ ☆ ☆ ☆ |

# Mood Tracker

| MONTH | | | | | | WEEK | | | |
|---|---|---|---|---|---|---|---|---|---|

| | MONDAY | TUESDAY | WEDNESDAY | THURSDAY | FRIDAY | SATURDAY | SUNDAY |
|---|---|---|---|---|---|---|---|
| **HAPPY** | | | | | | | |
| **NEUTRAL** | | | | | | | |
| **SAD** | | | | | | | |

| DAY | EMOTION | WHAT HAPPENED? | DAILY SCORE |
|---|---|---|---|
| MONDAY | | | ☆ ☆ ☆ ☆ ☆ |
| TUESDAY | | | ☆ ☆ ☆ ☆ ☆ |
| WEDNESDAY | | | ☆ ☆ ☆ ☆ ☆ |
| THURSDAY | | | ☆ ☆ ☆ ☆ ☆ |
| FRIDAY | | | ☆ ☆ ☆ ☆ ☆ |
| SATURDAY | | | ☆ ☆ ☆ ☆ ☆ |
| SUNDAY | | | ☆ ☆ ☆ ☆ ☆ |

# Mood Tracker

| MONTH | | | | | | WEEK | |
|---|---|---|---|---|---|---|---|

| | | | | | | | |
|---|---|---|---|---|---|---|---|
| HAPPY | | | | | | | |
| NEUTRAL | | | | | | | |
| SAD | | | | | | | |
| | MONDAY | TUESDAY | WEDNESDAY | THURSDAY | FRIDAY | SATURDAY | SUNDAY |

| DAY | EMOTION | WHAT HAPPENED? | DAILY SCORE |
|---|---|---|---|
| MONDAY | | | ☆ ☆ ☆ ☆ ☆ |
| TUESDAY | | | ☆ ☆ ☆ ☆ ☆ |
| WEDNESDAY | | | ☆ ☆ ☆ ☆ ☆ |
| THURSDAY | | | ★ ☆ ☆ ☆ ☆ |
| FRIDAY | | | ☆ ☆ ☆ ☆ ☆ |
| SATURDAY | | | ☆ ☆ ☆ ☆ ☆ |
| SUNDAY | | | ☆ ☆ ☆ ☆ ☆ |

# Mood Tracker

| MONTH | | | | | | | WEEK | | |
|---|---|---|---|---|---|---|---|---|---|

| | MONDAY | TUESDAY | WEDNESDAY | THURSDAY | FRIDAY | SATURDAY | SUNDAY |
|---|---|---|---|---|---|---|---|
| HAPPY | | | | | | | |
| NEUTRAL | | | | | | | |
| SAD | | | | | | | |

| DAY | EMOTION | WHAT HAPPENED? | DAILY SCORE |
|---|---|---|---|
| MONDAY | | | ☆ ☆ ☆ ☆ ☆ |
| TUESDAY | | | ☆ ☆ ☆ ☆ ☆ |
| WEDNESDAY | | | ☆ ☆ ☆ ☆ ☆ |
| THURSDAY | | | ☆ ☆ ☆ ☆ ☆ |
| FRIDAY | | | ☆ ☆ ☆ ☆ ☆ |
| SATURDAY | | | ☆ ☆ ☆ ☆ ☆ |
| SUNDAY | | | ☆ ☆ ☆ ☆ ☆ |

# Mood Tracker

| MONTH | | | | | WEEK | | |
|---|---|---|---|---|---|---|---|

| | MONDAY | TUESDAY | WEDNESDAY | THURSDAY | FRIDAY | SATURDAY | SUNDAY |
|---|---|---|---|---|---|---|---|
| HAPPY | | | | | | | |
| NEUTRAL | | | | | | | |
| SAD | | | | | | | |

| DAY | EMOTION | WHAT HAPPENED? | DAILY SCORE |
|---|---|---|---|
| MONDAY | | | ☆ ☆ ☆ ☆ ☆ |
| TUESDAY | | | ☆ ☆ ☆ ☆ ☆ |
| WEDNESDAY | | | ☆ ☆ ☆ ☆ ☆ |
| THURSDAY | | | ☆ ☆ ☆ ☆ ☆ |
| FRIDAY | | | ☆ ☆ ☆ ☆ ☆ |
| SATURDAY | | | ☆ ☆ ☆ ☆ ☆ |
| SUNDAY | | | ☆ ☆ ☆ ☆ ☆ |

# Mood Tracker

| MONTH | | | | | WEEK | |
|---|---|---|---|---|---|---|

| | MONDAY | TUESDAY | WEDNESDAY | THURSDAY | FRIDAY | SATURDAY | SUNDAY |
|---|---|---|---|---|---|---|---|
| HAPPY | | | | | | | |
| NEUTRAL | | | | | | | |
| SAD | | | | | | | |

| DAY | EMOTION | WHAT HAPPENED? | DAILY SCORE |
|---|---|---|---|
| MONDAY | | | ☆ ☆ ☆ ☆ ☆ |
| TUESDAY | | | ☆ ☆ ☆ ☆ ☆ |
| WEDNESDAY | | | ☆ ☆ ☆ ☆ ☆ |
| THURSDAY | | | ☆ ☆ ☆ ☆ ☆ |
| FRIDAY | | | ☆ ☆ ☆ ☆ ☆ |
| SATURDAY | | | ☆ ☆ ☆ ☆ ☆ |
| SUNDAY | | | ☆ ☆ ☆ ☆ ☆ |

# Mood Tracker

| MONTH | | | | | WEEK | | |
|---|---|---|---|---|---|---|---|

| | MONDAY | TUESDAY | WEDNESDAY | THURSDAY | FRIDAY | SATURDAY | SUNDAY |
|---|---|---|---|---|---|---|---|
| HAPPY | | | | | | | |
| NEUTRAL | | | | | | | |
| SAD | | | | | | | |

| DAY | EMOTION | WHAT HAPPENED? | DAILY SCORE |
|---|---|---|---|
| MONDAY | | | ☆ ☆ ☆ ☆ ☆ |
| TUESDAY | | | ☆ ☆ ☆ ☆ ☆ |
| WEDNESDAY | | | ☆ ☆ ☆ ☆ ☆ |
| THURSDAY | | | ☆ ☆ ☆ ☆ ☆ |
| FRIDAY | | | ☆ ☆ ☆ ☆ ☆ |
| SATURDAY | | | ☆ ☆ ☆ ☆ ☆ |
| SUNDAY | | | ☆ ☆ ☆ ☆ ☆ |

# Mood Tracker

| MONTH | | | | | WEEK | | | |
|---|---|---|---|---|---|---|---|---|

| | MONDAY | TUESDAY | WEDNESDAY | THURSDAY | FRIDAY | SATURDAY | SUNDAY |
|---|---|---|---|---|---|---|---|
| HAPPY | | | | | | | |
| NEUTRAL | | | | | | | |
| SAD | | | | | | | |

| DAY | EMOTION | WHAT HAPPENED? | DAILY SCORE |
|---|---|---|---|
| MONDAY | | | ☆ ☆ ☆ ☆ ☆ |
| TUESDAY | | | ☆ ☆ ☆ ☆ ☆ |
| WEDNESDAY | | | ☆ ☆ ☆ ☆ ☆ |
| THURSDAY | | | ☆ ☆ ☆ ☆ ☆ |
| FRIDAY | | | ☆ ☆ ☆ ☆ ☆ |
| SATURDAY | | | ☆ ☆ ☆ ☆ ☆ |
| SUNDAY | | | ☆ ☆ ☆ ☆ ☆ |

# Mood Tracker

| MONTH | | | | | | WEEK | | | |
|-------|---|---|---|---|---|------|---|---|---|

| | MONDAY | TUESDAY | WEDNESDAY | THURSDAY | FRIDAY | SATURDAY | SUNDAY |
|----------|--------|---------|-----------|----------|--------|----------|--------|
| HAPPY | | | | | | | |
| NEUTRAL | | | | | | | |
| SAD | | | | | | | |

| DAY | EMOTION | WHAT HAPPENED? | DAILY SCORE |
|-----|---------|----------------|-------------|
| MONDAY | | | ☆ ☆ ☆ ☆ ☆ |
| TUESDAY | | | ☆ ☆ ☆ ☆ ☆ |
| WEDNESDAY | | | ☆ ☆ ☆ ☆ ☆ |
| THURSDAY | | | ☆ ☆ ☆ ☆ ☆ |
| FRIDAY | | | ☆ ☆ ☆ ☆ ☆ |
| SATURDAY | | | ☆ ☆ ☆ ☆ ☆ |
| SUNDAY | | | ☆ ☆ ☆ ☆ ☆ |

# Mood Tracker

| MONTH | | | | | WEEK | | | |
|---|---|---|---|---|---|---|---|---|

| | MONDAY | TUESDAY | WEDNESDAY | THURSDAY | FRIDAY | SATURDAY | SUNDAY |
|---|---|---|---|---|---|---|---|
| **HAPPY** | | | | | | | |
| **NEUTRAL** | | | | | | | |
| **SAD** | | | | | | | |

| DAY | EMOTION | WHAT HAPPENED? | DAILY SCORE |
|---|---|---|---|
| MONDAY | | | ☆ ☆ ☆ ☆ ☆ |
| TUESDAY | | | ☆ ☆ ☆ ☆ ☆ |
| WEDNESDAY | | | ☆ ☆ ☆ ☆ ☆ |
| THURSDAY | | | ☆ ☆ ☆ ☆ ☆ |
| FRIDAY | | | ☆ ☆ ☆ ☆ ☆ |
| SATURDAY | | | ☆ ☆ ☆ ☆ ☆ |
| SUNDAY | | | ☆ ☆ ☆ ☆ ☆ |

# Mood Tracker

| MONTH | | WEEK | |
|-------|---|------|---|

| | MONDAY | TUESDAY | WEDNESDAY | THURSDAY | FRIDAY | SATURDAY | SUNDAY |
|---------|--------|---------|-----------|----------|--------|----------|--------|
| HAPPY | | | | | | | |
| NEUTRAL | | | | | | | |
| SAD | | | | | | | |

| DAY | EMOTION | WHAT HAPPENED? | DAILY SCORE |
|-----|---------|----------------|-------------|
| MONDAY | | | ☆ ☆ ☆ ☆ ☆ |
| TUESDAY | | | ☆ ☆ ☆ ☆ ☆ |
| WEDNESDAY | | | ☆ ☆ ☆ ☆ ☆ |
| THURSDAY | | | ☆ ☆ ☆ ☆ ☆ |
| FRIDAY | | | ☆ ☆ ☆ ☆ ☆ |
| SATURDAY | | | ☆ ☆ ☆ ☆ ☆ |
| SUNDAY | | | ☆ ☆ ☆ ☆ ☆ |

# Mood Tracker

| MONTH | | | | | | | WEEK | | | |
|---|---|---|---|---|---|---|---|---|---|---|

| | MONDAY | TUESDAY | WEDNESDAY | THURSDAY | FRIDAY | SATURDAY | SUNDAY |
|---|---|---|---|---|---|---|---|
| **HAPPY** | | | | | | | |
| **NEUTRAL** | | | | | | | |
| **SAD** | | | | | | | |

| DAY | EMOTION | WHAT HAPPENED? | DAILY SCORE |
|---|---|---|---|
| MONDAY | | | ☆ ☆ ☆ ☆ ☆ |
| TUESDAY | | | ☆ ☆ ☆ ☆ ☆ |
| WEDNESDAY | | | ☆ ☆ ☆ ☆ ☆ |
| THURSDAY | | | ☆ ☆ ☆ ☆ ☆ |
| FRIDAY | | | ☆ ☆ ☆ ☆ ☆ |
| SATURDAY | | | ☆ ☆ ☆ ☆ ☆ |
| SUNDAY | | | ☆ ☆ ☆ ☆ ☆ |

# Mood Tracker

| MONTH | | WEEK | |
|---|---|---|---|

| | MONDAY | TUESDAY | WEDNESDAY | THURSDAY | FRIDAY | SATURDAY | SUNDAY |
|---|---|---|---|---|---|---|---|
| HAPPY | | | | | | | |
| NEUTRAL | | | | | | | |
| SAD | | | | | | | |

| DAY | EMOTION | WHAT HAPPENED? | DAILY SCORE |
|---|---|---|---|
| MONDAY | | | ☆ ☆ ☆ ☆ ☆ |
| TUESDAY | | | ☆ ☆ ☆ ☆ ☆ |
| WEDNESDAY | | | ☆ ☆ ☆ ☆ ☆ |
| THURSDAY | | | ☆ ☆ ☆ ☆ ☆ |
| FRIDAY | | | ☆ ☆ ☆ ☆ ☆ |
| SATURDAY | | | ☆ ☆ ☆ ☆ ☆ |
| SUNDAY | | | ☆ ☆ ☆ ☆ ☆ |

# Mood Tracker

| MONTH | | | | | | WEEK | | |
|---|---|---|---|---|---|---|---|---|

| | MONDAY | TUESDAY | WEDNESDAY | THURSDAY | FRIDAY | SATURDAY | SUNDAY |
|---|---|---|---|---|---|---|---|
| **HAPPY** | | | | | | | |
| **NEUTRAL** | | | | | | | |
| **SAD** | | | | | | | |

| DAY | EMOTION | WHAT HAPPENED? | DAILY SCORE |
|---|---|---|---|
| MONDAY | | | ☆ ☆ ☆ ☆ ☆ |
| TUESDAY | | | ☆ ☆ ☆ ☆ ☆ |
| WEDNESDAY | | | ☆ ☆ ☆ ☆ ☆ |
| THURSDAY | | | ☆ ☆ ☆ ☆ ☆ |
| FRIDAY | | | ☆ ☆ ☆ ☆ ☆ |
| SATURDAY | | | ☆ ☆ ☆ ☆ ☆ |
| SUNDAY | | | ☆ ☆ ☆ ☆ ☆ |

# Mood Tracker

| MONTH | | WEEK | |
|---|---|---|---|

| | MONDAY | TUESDAY | WEDNESDAY | THURSDAY | FRIDAY | SATURDAY | SUNDAY |
|---|---|---|---|---|---|---|---|
| HAPPY | | | | | | | |
| NEUTRAL | | | | | | | |
| SAD | | | | | | | |

| DAY | EMOTION | WHAT HAPPENED? | DAILY SCORE |
|---|---|---|---|
| MONDAY | | | ☆ ☆ ☆ ☆ ☆ |
| TUESDAY | | | ☆ ☆ ☆ ☆ ☆ |
| WEDNESDAY | | | ☆ ☆ ☆ ☆ ☆ |
| THURSDAY | | | ★ ★ ★ ☆ ☆ |
| FRIDAY | | | ☆ ☆ ☆ ☆ ☆ |
| SATURDAY | | | ☆ ☆ ☆ ☆ ☆ |
| SUNDAY | | | ☆ ☆ ☆ ☆ ☆ |

# Mood Tracker

| MONTH | | | | | | | | WEEK | | |
|---|---|---|---|---|---|---|---|---|---|---|

| | MONDAY | TUESDAY | WEDNESDAY | THURSDAY | FRIDAY | SATURDAY | SUNDAY |
|---|---|---|---|---|---|---|---|
| HAPPY | | | | | | | |
| NEUTRAL | | | | | | | |
| SAD | | | | | | | |

| DAY | EMOTION | WHAT HAPPENED? | DAILY SCORE |
|---|---|---|---|
| MONDAY | | | ☆ ☆ ☆ ☆ ☆ |
| TUESDAY | | | ☆ ☆ ☆ ☆ ☆ |
| WEDNESDAY | | | ☆ ☆ ☆ ☆ ☆ |
| THURSDAY | | | ☆ ☆ ☆ ☆ ☆ |
| FRIDAY | | | ☆ ☆ ☆ ☆ ☆ |
| SATURDAY | | | ☆ ☆ ☆ ☆ ☆ |
| SUNDAY | | | ☆ ☆ ☆ ☆ ☆ |

# Mood Tracker

| MONTH | | WEEK | |
|---|---|---|---|

| | MONDAY | TUESDAY | WEDNESDAY | THURSDAY | FRIDAY | SATURDAY | SUNDAY |
|---|---|---|---|---|---|---|---|
| HAPPY | | | | | | | |
| NEUTRAL | | | | | | | |
| SAD | | | | | | | |

| DAY | EMOTION | WHAT HAPPENED? | DAILY SCORE |
|---|---|---|---|
| MONDAY | | | ☆ ☆ ☆ ☆ ☆ |
| TUESDAY | | | ☆ ☆ ☆ ☆ ☆ |
| WEDNESDAY | | | ☆ ☆ ☆ ☆ ☆ |
| THURSDAY | | | ☆ ☆ ☆ ☆ A |
| FRIDAY | | | ☆ ☆ ☆ ☆ ☆ |
| SATURDAY | | | ☆ ☆ ☆ ☆ ☆ |
| SUNDAY | | | ☆ ☆ ☆ ☆ ☆ |

# Mood Tracker

| MONTH | | | | | | | WEEK | | | |
|---|---|---|---|---|---|---|---|---|---|---|

| | MONDAY | TUESDAY | WEDNESDAY | THURSDAY | FRIDAY | SATURDAY | SUNDAY |
|---|---|---|---|---|---|---|---|
| **HAPPY** | | | | | | | |
| **NEUTRAL** | | | | | | | |
| **SAD** | | | | | | | |

| DAY | EMOTION | WHAT HAPPENED? | DAILY SCORE |
|---|---|---|---|
| MONDAY | | | ☆ ☆ ☆ ☆ ☆ |
| TUESDAY | | | ☆ ☆ ☆ ☆ ☆ |
| WEDNESDAY | | | ☆ ☆ ☆ ☆ ☆ |
| THURSDAY | | | ☆ ☆ ☆ ☆ ☆ |
| FRIDAY | | | ☆ ☆ ☆ ☆ ☆ |
| SATURDAY | | | ☆ ☆ ☆ ☆ ☆ |
| SUNDAY | | | ☆ ☆ ☆ ☆ ☆ |

# Mood Tracker

| MONTH | | | | | WEEK | | |
|---|---|---|---|---|---|---|---|

| | MONDAY | TUESDAY | WEDNESDAY | THURSDAY | FRIDAY | SATURDAY | SUNDAY |
|---|---|---|---|---|---|---|---|
| HAPPY | | | | | | | |
| NEUTRAL | | | | | | | |
| SAD | | | | | | | |

| DAY | EMOTION | WHAT HAPPENED? | DAILY SCORE |
|---|---|---|---|
| MONDAY | | | ☆ ☆ ☆ ☆ ☆ |
| TUESDAY | | | ☆ ☆ ☆ ☆ ☆ |
| WEDNESDAY | | | ☆ ☆ ☆ ☆ ☆ |
| THURSDAY | | | ★ ★ ★ ★ ☆ |
| FRIDAY | | | ☆ ☆ ☆ ☆ ☆ |
| SATURDAY | | | ☆ ☆ ☆ ☆ ☆ |
| SUNDAY | | | ☆ ☆ ☆ ☆ ☆ |

# Mood Tracker

| MONTH | | | | | WEEK | | | |
|---|---|---|---|---|---|---|---|---|

| | MONDAY | TUESDAY | WEDNESDAY | THURSDAY | FRIDAY | SATURDAY | SUNDAY |
|---|---|---|---|---|---|---|---|
| HAPPY | | | | | | | |
| NEUTRAL | | | | | | | |
| SAD | | | | | | | |

| DAY | EMOTION | WHAT HAPPENED? | DAILY SCORE |
|---|---|---|---|
| MONDAY | | | ☆ ☆ ☆ ☆ ☆ |
| TUESDAY | | | ☆ ☆ ☆ ☆ ☆ |
| WEDNESDAY | | | ☆ ☆ ☆ ☆ ☆ |
| THURSDAY | | | ☆ ☆ ☆ ☆ ☆ |
| FRIDAY | | | ☆ ☆ ☆ ☆ ☆ |
| SATURDAY | | | ☆ ☆ ☆ ☆ ☆ |
| SUNDAY | | | ☆ ☆ ☆ ☆ ☆ |

# Mood Tracker

| MONTH | | | | WEEK | | |
|-------|--|--|--|------|--|--|

| | MONDAY | TUESDAY | WEDNESDAY | THURSDAY | FRIDAY | SATURDAY | SUNDAY |
|-------|--------|---------|-----------|----------|--------|----------|--------|
| HAPPY | | | | | | | |
| NEUTRAL | | | | | | | |
| SAD | | | | | | | |

| DAY | EMOTION | WHAT HAPPENED? | DAILY SCORE |
|-----|---------|----------------|-------------|
| MONDAY | | | ☆ ☆ ☆ ☆ ☆ |
| TUESDAY | | | ☆ ☆ ☆ ☆ ☆ |
| WEDNESDAY | | | ☆ ☆ ☆ ☆ ☆ |
| THURSDAY | | | ☆ ☆ ☆ ☆ ☆ |
| FRIDAY | | | ☆ ☆ ☆ ☆ ☆ |
| SATURDAY | | | ☆ ☆ ☆ ☆ ☆ |
| SUNDAY | | | ☆ ☆ ☆ ☆ ☆ |

# Mood Tracker

| MONTH | | | | | WEEK | | | | |
|---|---|---|---|---|---|---|---|---|---|

| | MONDAY | TUESDAY | WEDNESDAY | THURSDAY | FRIDAY | SATURDAY | SUNDAY |
|---|---|---|---|---|---|---|---|
| HAPPY | | | | | | | |
| NEUTRAL | | | | | | | |
| SAD | | | | | | | |

| DAY | EMOTION | WHAT HAPPENED? | DAILY SCORE |
|---|---|---|---|
| MONDAY | | | ☆ ☆ ☆ ☆ ☆ |
| TUESDAY | | | ☆ ☆ ☆ ☆ ☆ |
| WEDNESDAY | | | ☆ ☆ ☆ ☆ ☆ |
| THURSDAY | | | ☆ ☆ ☆ ☆ ☆ |
| FRIDAY | | | ☆ ☆ ☆ ☆ ☆ |
| SATURDAY | | | ☆ ☆ ☆ ☆ ☆ |
| SUNDAY | | | ☆ ☆ ☆ ☆ ☆ |

# Mood Tracker

| MONTH | | | | | WEEK | |
|---|---|---|---|---|---|---|

| | MONDAY | TUESDAY | WEDNESDAY | THURSDAY | FRIDAY | SATURDAY | SUNDAY |
|---|---|---|---|---|---|---|---|
| HAPPY | | | | | | | |
| NEUTRAL | | | | | | | |
| SAD | | | | | | | |

| DAY | EMOTION | WHAT HAPPENED? | DAILY SCORE |
|---|---|---|---|
| MONDAY | | | ☆ ☆ ☆ ☆ ☆ |
| TUESDAY | | | ☆ ☆ ☆ ☆ ☆ |
| WEDNESDAY | | | ☆ ☆ ☆ ☆ ☆ |
| THURSDAY | | | ☆ ☆ ☆ ☆ ☆ |
| FRIDAY | | | ☆ ☆ ☆ ☆ ☆ |
| SATURDAY | | | ☆ ☆ ☆ ☆ ☆ |
| SUNDAY | | | ☆ ☆ ☆ ☆ ☆ |

# Mood Tracker

| MONTH | | | | | | | | WEEK | | | |
|---|---|---|---|---|---|---|---|---|---|---|---|

| | MONDAY | TUESDAY | WEDNESDAY | THURSDAY | FRIDAY | SATURDAY | SUNDAY |
|---|---|---|---|---|---|---|---|
| HAPPY | | | | | | | |
| NEUTRAL | | | | | | | |
| SAD | | | | | | | |

| DAY | EMOTION | WHAT HAPPENED? | DAILY SCORE |
|---|---|---|---|
| MONDAY | | | ☆ ☆ ☆ ☆ ☆ |
| TUESDAY | | | ☆ ☆ ☆ ☆ ☆ |
| WEDNESDAY | | | ☆ ☆ ☆ ☆ ☆ |
| THURSDAY | | | ☆ ☆ ☆ ☆ ☆ |
| FRIDAY | | | ☆ ☆ ☆ ☆ ☆ |
| SATURDAY | | | ☆ ☆ ☆ ☆ ☆ |
| SUNDAY | | | ☆ ☆ ☆ ☆ ☆ |

# Mood Tracker

| MONTH | | | WEEK | | |
|---|---|---|---|---|---|

|  | MONDAY | TUESDAY | WEDNESDAY | THURSDAY | FRIDAY | SATURDAY | SUNDAY |
|---|---|---|---|---|---|---|---|
| HAPPY | | | | | | | |
| NEUTRAL | | | | | | | |
| SAD | | | | | | | |

| DAY | EMOTION | WHAT HAPPENED? | DAILY SCORE |
|---|---|---|---|
| MONDAY | | | ☆ ☆ ☆ ☆ ☆ |
| TUESDAY | | | ☆ ☆ ☆ ☆ ☆ |
| WEDNESDAY | | | ☆ ☆ ☆ ☆ ☆ |
| THURSDAY | | | ☆ ☆ ☆ ☆ ☆ |
| FRIDAY | | | ☆ ☆ ☆ ☆ ☆ |
| SATURDAY | | | ☆ ☆ ☆ ☆ ☆ |
| SUNDAY | | | ☆ ☆ ☆ ☆ ☆ |

# Mood Tracker

| MONTH | | | | WEEK | | |
|---|---|---|---|---|---|---|

| | MONDAY | TUESDAY | WEDNESDAY | THURSDAY | FRIDAY | SATURDAY | SUNDAY |
|---|---|---|---|---|---|---|---|
| HAPPY | | | | | | | |
| NEUTRAL | | | | | | | |
| SAD | | | | | | | |

| DAY | EMOTION | WHAT HAPPENED? | DAILY SCORE |
|---|---|---|---|
| MONDAY | | | ☆ ☆ ☆ ☆ ☆ |
| TUESDAY | | | ☆ ☆ ☆ ☆ ☆ |
| WEDNESDAY | | | ☆ ☆ ☆ ☆ ☆ |
| THURSDAY | | | ☆ ☆ ☆ ☆ ☆ |
| FRIDAY | | | ☆ ☆ ☆ ☆ ☆ |
| SATURDAY | | | ☆ ☆ ☆ ☆ ☆ |
| SUNDAY | | | ☆ ☆ ☆ ☆ ☆ |

# Mood Tracker

| MONTH | | WEEK | |
|---|---|---|---|

| | MONDAY | TUESDAY | WEDNESDAY | THURSDAY | FRIDAY | SATURDAY | SUNDAY |
|---|---|---|---|---|---|---|---|
| HAPPY | | | | | | | |
| NEUTRAL | | | | | | | |
| SAD | | | | | | | |

| DAY | EMOTION | WHAT HAPPENED? | DAILY SCORE |
|---|---|---|---|
| MONDAY | | | ☆ ☆ ☆ ☆ ☆ |
| TUESDAY | | | ☆ ☆ ☆ ☆ ☆ |
| WEDNESDAY | | | ☆ ☆ ☆ ☆ ☆ |
| THURSDAY | | | ☆ ☆ ☆ ☆ ☆ |
| FRIDAY | | | ☆ ☆ ☆ ☆ ☆ |
| SATURDAY | | | ☆ ☆ ☆ ☆ ☆ |
| SUNDAY | | | ☆ ☆ ☆ ☆ ☆ |

# Mood Tracker

| MONTH | | | | | | WEEK | | | |
|---|---|---|---|---|---|---|---|---|---|

| | | | | | | | | | |
|---|---|---|---|---|---|---|---|---|---|
| HAPPY | | | | | | | | | |
| NEUTRAL | | | | | | | | | |
| SAD | | | | | | | | | |
| | MONDAY | TUESDAY | WEDNESDAY | THURSDAY | FRIDAY | SATURDAY | SUNDAY | | |

| DAY | EMOTION | WHAT HAPPENED? | DAILY SCORE |
|---|---|---|---|
| MONDAY | | | ☆ ☆ ☆ ☆ ☆ |
| TUESDAY | | | ☆ ☆ ☆ ☆ ☆ |
| WEDNESDAY | | | ☆ ☆ ☆ ☆ ☆ |
| THURSDAY | | | ☆ ☆ ☆ ☆ ☆ |
| FRIDAY | | | ☆ ☆ ☆ ☆ ☆ |
| SATURDAY | | | ☆ ☆ ☆ ☆ ☆ |
| SUNDAY | | | ☆ ☆ ☆ ☆ ☆ |

# Mood Tracker

| MONTH | | | | WEEK | | | |
|---|---|---|---|---|---|---|---|

| | MONDAY | TUESDAY | WEDNESDAY | THURSDAY | FRIDAY | SATURDAY | SUNDAY |
|---|---|---|---|---|---|---|---|
| HAPPY | | | | | | | |
| NEUTRAL | | | | | | | |
| SAD | | | | | | | |

| DAY | EMOTION | WHAT HAPPENED? | DAILY SCORE |
|---|---|---|---|
| MONDAY | | | ☆ ☆ ☆ ☆ ☆ |
| TUESDAY | | | ☆ ☆ ☆ ☆ ☆ |
| WEDNESDAY | | | ☆ ☆ ☆ ☆ ☆ |
| THURSDAY | | | ☆ ☆ ☆ ☆ ☆ |
| FRIDAY | | | ☆ ☆ ☆ ☆ ☆ |
| SATURDAY | | | ☆ ☆ ☆ ☆ ☆ |
| SUNDAY | | | ☆ ☆ ☆ ☆ ☆ |

# Mood Tracker

| MONTH | | | | | | | WEEK | |
|---|---|---|---|---|---|---|---|---|

| | MONDAY | TUESDAY | WEDNESDAY | THURSDAY | FRIDAY | SATURDAY | SUNDAY |
|---|---|---|---|---|---|---|---|
| **HAPPY** | | | | | | | |
| **NEUTRAL** | | | | | | | |
| **SAD** | | | | | | | |

| DAY | EMOTION | WHAT HAPPENED? | DAILY SCORE |
|---|---|---|---|
| MONDAY | | | ★★★★☆ |
| TUESDAY | | | ★★★★☆ |
| WEDNESDAY | | | ★★★★☆ |
| THURSDAY | | | ★★★★☆ |
| FRIDAY | | | ★★★★☆ |
| SATURDAY | | | ★★★★☆ |
| SUNDAY | | | ★★★★☆ |

# Mood Tracker

| MONTH | | WEEK | |
|---|---|---|---|

| | MONDAY | TUESDAY | WEDNESDAY | THURSDAY | FRIDAY | SATURDAY | SUNDAY |
|---|---|---|---|---|---|---|---|
| HAPPY | | | | | | | |
| NEUTRAL | | | | | | | |
| SAD | | | | | | | |

| DAY. | EMOTION | WHAT HAPPENED? | DAILY SCORE |
|---|---|---|---|
| MONDAY | | | ☆ ☆ ☆ ☆ ☆ |
| TUESDAY | | | ☆ ☆ ☆ ☆ ☆ |
| WEDNESDAY | | | ☆ ☆ ☆ ☆ ☆ |
| THURSDAY | | | ☆ ☆ ☆ ☆ ★ |
| FRIDAY | | | ☆ ☆ ☆ ☆ ☆ |
| SATURDAY | | | ☆ ☆ ☆ ☆ ☆ |
| SUNDAY | | | ☆ ☆ ☆ ☆ ☆ |

# Mood Tracker

| MONTH | | | | | | WEEK | | | | | |
|---|---|---|---|---|---|---|---|---|---|---|---|

| | MONDAY | TUESDAY | WEDNESDAY | THURSDAY | FRIDAY | SATURDAY | SUNDAY |
|---|---|---|---|---|---|---|---|
| HAPPY | | | | | | | |
| NEUTRAL | | | | | | | |
| SAD | | | | | | | |

| DAY | EMOTION | WHAT HAPPENED? | DAILY SCORE |
|---|---|---|---|
| MONDAY | | | ☆ ☆ ☆ ☆ ☆ |
| TUESDAY | | | ☆ ☆ ☆ ☆ ☆ |
| WEDNESDAY | | | ☆ ☆ ☆ ☆ ☆ |
| THURSDAY | | | ☆ ☆ ☆ ☆ ☆ |
| FRIDAY | | | ☆ ☆ ☆ ☆ ☆ |
| SATURDAY | | | ☆ ☆ ☆ ☆ ☆ |
| SUNDAY | | | ☆ ☆ ☆ ☆ ☆ |

# Mood Tracker

| MONTH | | | | | WEEK | | |
|---|---|---|---|---|---|---|---|

| | MONDAY | TUESDAY | WEDNESDAY | THURSDAY | FRIDAY | SATURDAY | SUNDAY |
|---|---|---|---|---|---|---|---|
| HAPPY | | | | | | | |
| NEUTRAL | | | | | | | |
| SAD | | | | | | | |

| DAY | EMOTION | WHAT HAPPENED? | DAILY SCORE |
|---|---|---|---|
| MONDAY | | | ☆ ☆ ☆ ☆ ☆ |
| TUESDAY | | | ☆ ☆ ☆ ☆ ☆ |
| WEDNESDAY | | | ☆ ☆ ☆ ☆ ☆ |
| THURSDAY | | | ☆ ☆ ☆ ☆ ☆ |
| FRIDAY | | | ☆ ☆ ☆ ☆ ☆ |
| SATURDAY | | | ☆ ☆ ☆ ☆ ☆ |
| SUNDAY | | | ☆ ☆ ☆ ☆ ☆ |

# Mood Tracker

| MONTH | | | | | | | WEEK | | |
|-------|---|---|---|---|---|---|---|---|---|

| | MONDAY | TUESDAY | WEDNESDAY | THURSDAY | FRIDAY | SATURDAY | SUNDAY |
|-------|--------|---------|-----------|----------|--------|----------|--------|
| HAPPY | | | | | | | |
| NEUTRAL | | | | | | | |
| SAD | | | | | | | |

| DAY | EMOTION | WHAT HAPPENED? | DAILY SCORE |
|-----|---------|----------------|-------------|
| MONDAY | | | ☆ ☆ ☆ ☆ ☆ |
| TUESDAY | | | ☆ ☆ ☆ ☆ ☆ |
| WEDNESDAY | | | ☆ ☆ ☆ ☆ ☆ |
| THURSDAY | | | ☆ ☆ ☆ ☆ ☆ |
| FRIDAY | | | ☆ ☆ ☆ ☆ ☆ |
| SATURDAY | | | ☆ ☆ ☆ ☆ ☆ |
| SUNDAY | | | ☆ ☆ ☆ ☆ ☆ |

# Mood Tracker

| MONTH | | | | WEEK | | | |
|-------|---|---|---|------|---|---|---|

| | | | | | | | |
|------|--------|---------|-----------|----------|--------|----------|--------|
| HAPPY | | | | | | | |
| NEUTRAL | | | | | | | |
| SAD | | | | | | | |
| | MONDAY | TUESDAY | WEDNESDAY | THURSDAY | FRIDAY | SATURDAY | SUNDAY |

| DAY | EMOTION | WHAT HAPPENED? | DAILY SCORE |
|-----|---------|----------------|-------------|
| MONDAY | | | ☆ ☆ ☆ ☆ ☆ |
| TUESDAY | | | ☆ ☆ ☆ ☆ ☆ |
| WEDNESDAY | | | ☆ ☆ ☆ ☆ ☆ |
| THURSDAY | | | ☆ ☆ ☆ ☆ ☆ |
| FRIDAY | | | ☆ ☆ ☆ ☆ ☆ |
| SATURDAY | | | ☆ ☆ ☆ ☆ ☆ |
| SUNDAY | | | ☆ ☆ ☆ ☆ ☆ |

# Mood Tracker

| MONTH | | | | | | | | | WEEK | |
|---|---|---|---|---|---|---|---|---|---|---|

| | MONDAY | TUESDAY | WEDNESDAY | THURSDAY | FRIDAY | SATURDAY | SUNDAY |
|---|---|---|---|---|---|---|---|
| **HAPPY** | | | | | | | |
| **NEUTRAL** | | | | | | | |
| **SAD** | | | | | | | |

| DAY | EMOTION | WHAT HAPPENED? | DAILY SCORE |
|---|---|---|---|
| MONDAY | | | ☆☆☆☆☆ |
| TUESDAY | | | ☆☆☆☆☆ |
| WEDNESDAY | | | ☆☆☆☆☆ |
| THURSDAY | | | ☆☆☆☆☆ |
| FRIDAY | | | ☆☆☆☆☆ |
| SATURDAY | | | ☆☆☆☆☆ |
| SUNDAY | | | ☆☆☆☆☆ |

# Mood Tracker

| MONTH | | | | WEEK | | | |
|---|---|---|---|---|---|---|---|

| | MONDAY | TUESDAY | WEDNESDAY | THURSDAY | FRIDAY | SATURDAY | SUNDAY |
|---|---|---|---|---|---|---|---|
| HAPPY | | | | | | | |
| NEUTRAL | | | | | | | |
| SAD | | | | | | | |

| DAY | EMOTION | WHAT HAPPENED? | DAILY SCORE |
|---|---|---|---|
| MONDAY | | | ☆ ☆ ☆ ☆ ☆ |
| TUESDAY | | | ☆ ☆ ☆ ☆ ☆ |
| WEDNESDAY | | | ☆ ☆ ☆ ☆ ☆ |
| THURSDAY | | | ☆ ☆ ☆ ☆ ☆ |
| FRIDAY | | | ☆ ☆ ☆ ☆ ☆ |
| SATURDAY | | | ☆ ☆ ☆ ☆ ☆ |
| SUNDAY | | | ☆ ☆ ☆ ☆ ☆ |

# Mood Tracker

| MONTH | | | | | | | | WEEK | |
|---|---|---|---|---|---|---|---|---|---|

| | MONDAY | TUESDAY | WEDNESDAY | THURSDAY | FRIDAY | SATURDAY | SUNDAY |
|---|---|---|---|---|---|---|---|
| HAPPY | | | | | | | |
| NEUTRAL | | | | | | | |
| SAD | | | | | | | |

| DAY | EMOTION | WHAT HAPPENED? | DAILY SCORE |
|---|---|---|---|
| MONDAY | | | ☆ ☆ ☆ ☆ ☆ |
| TUESDAY | | | ☆ ☆ ☆ ☆ ☆ |
| WEDNESDAY | | | ☆ ☆ ☆ ☆ ☆ |
| THURSDAY | | | ☆ ☆ ☆ ☆ ☆ |
| FRIDAY | | | ☆ ☆ ☆ ☆ ☆ |
| SATURDAY | | | ☆ ☆ ☆ ☆ ☆ |
| SUNDAY | | | ☆ ☆ ☆ ☆ ☆ |

# Mood Tracker

| MONTH | | | | | | | WEEK | | |
|---|---|---|---|---|---|---|---|---|---|

| | | | | | | | |
|---|---|---|---|---|---|---|---|
| HAPPY | | | | | | | |
| NEUTRAL | | | | | | | |
| SAD | | | | | | | |
| | MONDAY | TUESDAY | WEDNESDAY | THURSDAY | FRIDAY | SATURDAY | SUNDAY |

| DAY | EMOTION | WHAT HAPPENED? | DAILY SCORE |
|---|---|---|---|
| MONDAY | | | ☆ ☆ ☆ ☆ ☆ |
| TUESDAY | | | ☆ ☆ ☆ ☆ ☆ |
| WEDNESDAY | | | ☆ ☆ ☆ ☆ ☆ |
| THURSDAY | | | ☆ ☆ ☆ ☆ ☆ |
| FRIDAY | | | ☆ ☆ ☆ ☆ ☆ |
| SATURDAY | | | ☆ ☆ ☆ ☆ ☆ |
| SUNDAY | | | ☆ ☆ ☆ ☆ ☆ |

# Mood Tracker

| MONTH | | | | | | | WEEK | | | |
|---|---|---|---|---|---|---|---|---|---|---|

| | MONDAY | TUESDAY | WEDNESDAY | THURSDAY | FRIDAY | SATURDAY | SUNDAY |
|---|---|---|---|---|---|---|---|
| HAPPY | | | | | | | |
| NEUTRAL | | | | | | | |
| SAD | | | | | | | |

| DAY | EMOTION | WHAT HAPPENED? | DAILY SCORE |
|---|---|---|---|
| MONDAY | | | ☆ ☆ ☆ ☆ ☆ |
| TUESDAY | | | ☆ ☆ ☆ ☆ ☆ |
| WEDNESDAY | | | ☆ ☆ ☆ ☆ ☆ |
| THURSDAY | | | ☆ ☆ ☆ ☆ ☆ |
| FRIDAY | | | ☆ ☆ ☆ ☆ ☆ |
| SATURDAY | | | ☆ ☆ ☆ ☆ ☆ |
| SUNDAY | | | ☆ ☆ ☆ ☆ ☆ |

# Mood Tracker

| MONTH | | WEEK | |
|---|---|---|---|

| | MONDAY | TUESDAY | WEDNESDAY | THURSDAY | FRIDAY | SATURDAY | SUNDAY |
|---|---|---|---|---|---|---|---|
| **HAPPY** | | | | | | | |
| **NEUTRAL** | | | | | | | |
| **SAD** | | | | | | | |

| DAY | EMOTION | WHAT HAPPENED? | DAILY SCORE |
|---|---|---|---|
| MONDAY | | | ☆ ☆ ☆ ☆ ☆ |
| TUESDAY | | | ☆ ☆ ☆ ☆ ☆ |
| WEDNESDAY | | | ☆ ☆ ☆ ☆ ☆ |
| THURSDAY | | | ☆ ☆ ☆ ☆ ☆ |
| FRIDAY | | | ☆ ☆ ☆ ☆ ☆ |
| SATURDAY | | | ☆ ☆ ☆ ☆ ☆ |
| SUNDAY | | | ☆ ☆ ☆ ☆ ☆ |

# Mood Tracker

| MONTH | | | WEEK | |
|---|---|---|---|---|

| | MONDAY | TUESDAY | WEDNESDAY | THURSDAY | FRIDAY | SATURDAY | SUNDAY |
|---|---|---|---|---|---|---|---|
| **HAPPY** | | | | | | | |
| **NEUTRAL** | | | | | | | |
| **SAD** | | | | | | | |

| DAY | EMOTION | WHAT HAPPENED? | DAILY SCORE |
|---|---|---|---|
| MONDAY | | | ☆ ☆ ☆ ☆ ☆ |
| TUESDAY | | | ☆ ☆ ☆ ☆ ☆ |
| WEDNESDAY | | | ☆ ☆ ☆ ☆ ☆ |
| THURSDAY | | | ☆ ☆ ☆ ☆ ☆ |
| FRIDAY | | | ☆ ☆ ☆ ☆ ☆ |
| SATURDAY | | | ☆ ☆ ☆ ☆ ☆ |
| SUNDAY | | | ☆ ☆ ☆ ☆ ☆ |

# Mood Tracker

| MONTH | | | | | WEEK | | | |
|---|---|---|---|---|---|---|---|---|

| | MONDAY | TUESDAY | WEDNESDAY | THURSDAY | FRIDAY | SATURDAY | SUNDAY |
|---|---|---|---|---|---|---|---|
| HAPPY | | | | | | | |
| NEUTRAL | | | | | | | |
| SAD | | | | | | | |

| DAY | EMOTION | WHAT HAPPENED? | DAILY SCORE |
|---|---|---|---|
| MONDAY | | | ☆ ☆ ☆ ☆ ☆ |
| TUESDAY | | | ☆ ☆ ☆ ☆ ☆ |
| WEDNESDAY | | | ☆ ☆ ☆ ☆ ☆ |
| THURSDAY | | | ☆ ☆ ☆ ☆ ☆ |
| FRIDAY | | | ☆ ☆ ☆ ☆ ☆ |
| SATURDAY | | | ☆ ☆ ☆ ☆ ☆ |
| SUNDAY | | | ☆ ☆ ☆ ☆ ☆ |

# Mood Tracker

| MONTH | | | | | | WEEK | | | |
|-------|--|--|--|--|--|------|--|--|--|

| | MONDAY | TUESDAY | WEDNESDAY | THURSDAY | FRIDAY | SATURDAY | SUNDAY |
|--------|--------|---------|-----------|----------|--------|----------|--------|
| HAPPY | | | | | | | |
| NEUTRAL | | | | | | | |
| SAD | | | | | | | |

| DAY | EMOTION | WHAT HAPPENED? | DAILY SCORE |
|-----|---------|----------------|-------------|
| MONDAY | | | ☆ ☆ ☆ ☆ ☆ |
| TUESDAY | | | ☆ ☆ ☆ ☆ ☆ |
| WEDNESDAY | | | ☆ ☆ ☆ ☆ ☆ |
| THURSDAY | | | ☆ ☆ ☆ ☆ ☆ |
| FRIDAY | | | ☆ ☆ ☆ ☆ ☆ |
| SATURDAY | | | ☆ ☆ ☆ ☆ ☆ |
| SUNDAY | | | ☆ ☆ ☆ ☆ ☆ |

# Mood Tracker

| MONTH | | | | WEEK | | | |
|---|---|---|---|---|---|---|---|

| | MONDAY | TUESDAY | WEDNESDAY | THURSDAY | FRIDAY | SATURDAY | SUNDAY |
|---|---|---|---|---|---|---|---|
| HAPPY | | | | | | | |
| NEUTRAL | | | | | | | |
| SAD | | | | | | | |

| DAY | EMOTION | WHAT HAPPENED? | DAILY SCORE |
|---|---|---|---|
| MONDAY | | | ☆ ☆ ☆ ☆ ☆ |
| TUESDAY | | | ☆ ☆ ☆ ☆ ☆ |
| WEDNESDAY | | | ☆ ☆ ☆ ☆ ☆ |
| THURSDAY | | | A A A A A |
| FRIDAY | | | ☆ ☆ ☆ ☆ ☆ |
| SATURDAY | | | ☆ ☆ ☆ ☆ ☆ |
| SUNDAY | | | ☆ ☆ ☆ ☆ ☆ |

# Mood Tracker

| MONTH | | | | | | WEEK | | |
|---|---|---|---|---|---|---|---|---|

| | MONDAY | TUESDAY | WEDNESDAY | THURSDAY | FRIDAY | SATURDAY | SUNDAY |
|---|---|---|---|---|---|---|---|
| HAPPY | | | | | | | |
| NEUTRAL | | | | | | | |
| SAD | | | | | | | |

| DAY | EMOTION | WHAT HAPPENED? | DAILY SCORE |
|---|---|---|---|
| MONDAY | | | ☆ ☆ ☆ ☆ ☆ |
| TUESDAY | | | ☆ ☆ ☆ ☆ ☆ |
| WEDNESDAY | | | ☆ ☆ ☆ ☆ ☆ |
| THURSDAY | | | ☆ ☆ ☆ ☆ ☆ |
| FRIDAY | | | ☆ ☆ ☆ ☆ ☆ |
| SATURDAY | | | ☆ ☆ ☆ ☆ ☆ |
| SUNDAY | | | ☆ ☆ ☆ ☆ ☆ |

# Mood Tracker

| MONTH | | | WEEK | | |
|---|---|---|---|---|---|

| | MONDAY | TUESDAY | WEDNESDAY | THURSDAY | FRIDAY | SATURDAY | SUNDAY |
|---|---|---|---|---|---|---|---|
| HAPPY | | | | | | | |
| NEUTRAL | | | | | | | |
| SAD | | | | | | | |

| DAY | EMOTION | WHAT HAPPENED? | DAILY SCORE |
|---|---|---|---|
| MONDAY | | | ☆ ☆ ☆ ☆ ☆ |
| TUESDAY | | | ☆ ☆ ☆ ☆ ☆ |
| WEDNESDAY | | | ☆ ☆ ☆ ☆ ☆ |
| THURSDAY | | | ☆ ★ ☆ ☆ ☆ |
| FRIDAY | | | ☆ ☆ ☆ ☆ ☆ |
| SATURDAY | | | ☆ ☆ ☆ ☆ ☆ |
| SUNDAY | | | ☆ ☆ ☆ ☆ ☆ |

# Mood Tracker

| MONTH | | | | | | | | WEEK | | | |
|---|---|---|---|---|---|---|---|---|---|---|---|

| | | | | | | | | |
|---|---|---|---|---|---|---|---|---|
| HAPPY | | | | | | | | |
| NEUTRAL | | | | | | | | |
| SAD | | | | | | | | |
| | MONDAY | TUESDAY | WEDNESDAY | THURSDAY | FRIDAY | SATURDAY | SUNDAY | |

| DAY | EMOTION | WHAT HAPPENED? | DAILY SCORE |
|---|---|---|---|
| MONDAY | | | ☆ ☆ ☆ ☆ ☆ |
| TUESDAY | | | ☆ ☆ ☆ ☆ ☆ |
| WEDNESDAY | | | ☆ ☆ ☆ ☆ ☆ |
| THURSDAY | | | ☆ ☆ ☆ ☆ ☆ |
| FRIDAY | | | ☆ ☆ ☆ ☆ ☆ |
| SATURDAY | | | ☆ ☆ ☆ ☆ ☆ |
| SUNDAY | | | ☆ ☆ ☆ ☆ ☆ |